CHEMICAL COURAGE

REFRAMING THE BULLY WITHIN FOR A HEALTHIER WORLD

JAMES ZEIGLER

Copyright ©2024 by James Zeigler

All rights reserved.

No portion of this book may be reproduced in any form without written permission from the author, except as permitted by U.S. copyright law.

This publication is designed to provide accurate and authoritative information in regard to the subject matter covered. It is sold with the understanding that the author is engaged in rendering legal, investment, accounting or other professional services. While the author has used their best efforts in preparing this book, they make no representations or warranties with respect to the accuracy or completeness of the contents of this book and specifically disclaim any implied warranties of merchantability or fitness for a particular purpose. No warranty may be created or extended by sales representatives or written sales materials. The advice and strategies contained herein may not be suitable for your situation. You should consult with a professional when appropriate. The author shall not be liable for any loss of profit or any other commercial damages, including but not limited to special, incidental, consequential, personal, or other damages.

Illustrations by Wesley Spurgeon
Cover and Interior compiled by Descendant Publishing LLC

ISBN 979-8-9918792-0-0 (Paperback)
ISBN 979-8-9918792-1-7 (Ebook)

First edition November 2024

Brendie, you were my editor-in-chief, my biggest supporter, and you gave me the gift of time to fulfill a dream of writing a book one day. We did it! Thank you and thank God.

Praise for Chemical Courage

Are you tired of feeling bullied at work or at home? Do you long for a way to reclaim your power and dignity? James Zeigler's 'Chemical Courage: Reframing the Bully Within for a Healthier World' is the book you've been waiting for.

As a cofounder of Dream Leader Institute, I'm excited to recommend this powerful exploration of workplace and personal bullying. Zeigler doesn't just identify problems; he offers a pathway to transformation and hope. His insights on confronting our 'inner bully' and fostering emotional intelligence align perfectly with our mission to help people reach their full potential.

This book will show you that you're not alone in your struggles. It provides practical strategies to build your inner being and create positive change in your life. Whether you're dealing with workplace toxicity or personal relationships challenges, 'Chemical Courage' offers the tools to become the hero of your own story.

Prepare to have your eyes opened and your heart touched. This is essential reading for anyone ready to break free from the cycle of bullying and step into their greatest self.

Dr. Clifford J Fisher
Co-founder of Dream Leader Institute

Contents

Foreword	VII
ENTITY ONE: INTENTION	
My "Why"	3
Know your Enemy Know your Friend	5
Kindergarten to the C-Suite	9
Normal Reactions to Abnormal Situations	21
When God Shows Up to Coach Mr. Resilience	23
See the Church See the Steeple...	29
Crooked Road Ahead	35
Presence Pause	37
Some Science to Ponder	41
Call to Action!	45
ENTITY TWO: INSIGHTS	
1. Minister of Defense – Injured Reserve List	53
2. Snowed in with Dracula	59
3. Scrambled Chicken Embryos on Ice	69
4. Coming Clean	77
Belle's Diary: Entry One	91
5. Purple Polka-Dotted – Back to School	93

6. Blurred "Code" Grey Lines	103
Belle's Diary: Entry Two	114
7. Leaving the Scene of a Crime	117
8. Do You Hear What I Hear?	123
9. Candy and Cavities	131
10. Too Sexy for My Shirt	145
Belle's Diary Entry 3	155
11. Desperate Times – Drastic Measures	157
Belle's Diary Entry 4	167
12. Quarterbacking	169
13. Burgers, Babble, and the Last Supper	177
Belle's Diary Entry 5	193
14. Gathering Grief	197
15. Going Through the Hoops	205
16. Return Recipe to Sender	219
17. Road Trip and Roadside Stop	225
18. The Rest of the Story	231
19. Mine!	245
20. Birdhouse Bullies	257
21. Burned the Candle-But Not Both Ends	265
22. The Long Trip Home	281

ENTITY THREE: INDIVIDUAL IMPLEMENTATION

Author's Note	291
Worksheets	295
About the Author	301

Foreword

It has been my pleasure to know and occasionally work with James Zeigler over the last nearly 10 years both as a colleague and then a friend. As a clinical psychologist and neuropsychologist, as well as the Chief of a rather large mental health group, I gleaned from his leadership skills, as well as appreciate his sincere and honest friendship. Furthermore, I have studied and have a strong understanding of resilience and how it can help my patients.

Resilience, from a psychological perspective, is very useful in bringing patients back from a place of helplessness. However, James has given me a view of "the other side" of resilience. He may have learned something from me over the years regarding resilience but I have learned even more about his journey, the downfalls of resilience and why both sides of resilience are important.

When I first met James I was impressed with his organizational abilities, his professional stance, and impressive leadership skills. I knew one or two of my staff had obtained leadership mentoring with him and one mentioned loving their experience working and learning "at the feet of the master". I must mention that I was envious of their ability to work with him. We would all benefit from his mentoring. With that said, I am very happy with our friendship and his honesty.

I remember the day our personal relationship started; he was getting off the elevator and I shared that our boss had mentioned him in a very positive light during a recent leadership meeting that he was unable to attend. I remember his surprised look and his admission that he was not what he seemed to be, that he was not feeling successful. I was impressed with his honesty and his willingness to be open with a colleague. I was also confused by his admission given he did not appear, in any way, to be unsuccessful in his job. The relationship that formed afterwards has been and continues to be a relationship of growth, kindness and mutual respect.

With that said, I highly recommend his book, appreciate his perspective and feel he has insights about how to walk a more fulfilling path. I recognize his life struggles led him to this moment in time. He has found peace, true faith and a clear vision of a process to help others meet their moment in time, their faith, and rid themselves of their bullies within. The holy trinity is an amazing concept by which to share his knowledge. I know each reader will gain insights and grow as a result of their reading about James' journey and insights. You will learn you are not alone, that there is a way to find yourself and a path to live a better life.

Dr. Elizabeth M. Stanczak, Ph.D
Clinical Psychologist, Neuropsychologist
Retired

ENTITY ONE
INTENTION

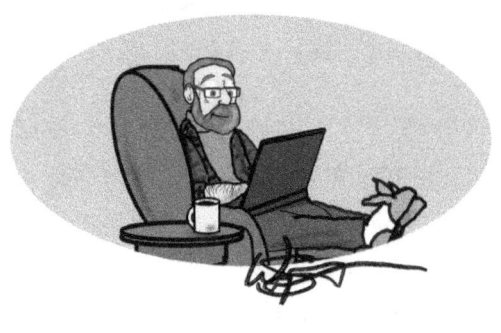

My "Why"

Hello, my name is James, and I am a bully.

This may sound like the beginning of a twelve-step program—Bullies Anonymous. I could also have begun with, "Hello, my name is James, aka 'Mr. Resilience.'" I rode that dark horse named resilience to the point of near death. I wore that medal of tolerance proudly, striving for it like Olympic gold. I ate, slept, and drank that cultish Kool-Aid. I was fooled into false fulfillment when people called me "Mr. Resilience." Yeah, baby!

The canvas of our lives will be adorned by our journey. It will be painted with the odds, coincidences, fate, second chances or even the do-overs. It will show how much downright amazing, miraculous grace was extended to us in our human existence! The Psalmist wrote that there is "...a lamp unto my path and a light unto my feet." I hope that by reframing resilience for myself, and possibly for many others, will result in us all becoming refined works of art at the Master's hand.

Life is beautiful and complicated enough. We will be accounted for how we lived it. Why must we *hurt one another*? The people we meet and treat are gifts to and for us.

Recently, a mentee told me something I had said to him years ago that impacted him. I have a habit of writing a scripture or inspirational thought at the top of my daily planner. It guides me. I had no idea how my personal compass could be so powerfully predictive for someone else. He told me I said,

"The road of life is full of twists and turns. What matters is who is in the driver's seat and how good of a passenger we are."

The book is divided into three entities, just like the Holy Trinity:

ENTITY ONE: INTENTION (Me)

ENTITY TWO: INSIGHTS (Others)

ENTITY THREE: INDIVIDUAL IMPLEMENTATION (You)

Know your Enemy
Know your Friend

An enemy's goal is to seek, kill, and destroy. A friend builds and protects. What is *resilience*, and why am I writing to clarify something in our language I observed that society has come to adore in leaders? Is it friend or foe? Could this be a scarlet letter R of sorts? Have you ever been just a little curious yourself? A lot of definitions exist, but at its core, resilience can be thought of as:

> *An expectation that when an outside force is imposed upon a substance or material, there is a measure of the amount of time it takes to <u>return to an original shape or function</u>.*

Crush a plastic water bottle in your hand. Does it completely go back to being a water bottle? Maybe with time. Humans don't have this physical and/or mental ability. Why do we use this word to describe human strength in the face of unnecessary adversity? Do we really need to be resilient in the paths of bullying? Is the onus on the right party? The purpose of this book is to reframe our awareness and to help us find presence. In the moment, while discovering healthy ways to shift the bullseye off each other's backs, we can be empowered to place it on the act of bullying rightly. Our actions must be carefully exercised in pure curiosity to achieve greatness with genuine kindness in the workplace and in our lives. Why lose some days and win others? How about we win them all?

Philippians 3:12-16. "It's not that I've already reached the goal or have already completed the course. But I run to win that which Jesus Christ has already won for me."

We bear the wounds. We don't return to normal like plastic.

I bet you can think of some bullying variations from childhood to old age--the *disorder* just seems to be engrained in our culture. In fact, the National Institute of Health considers bullying a public health issue.

Did you bully yourself or others? Were you bullied, or both?

You may be seasoned enough to remember the television show *The Little Rascals*. Not all bullies look or act as obvious as "Butch" in his black leather jacket, backward-worn black ball cap and no-fear threats. Passive aggression is a tough skill, but it is a deadly combination for a smart and skilled bully to cover their tracks while they undermine, showboat, or withhold information to broker their power in relationships. Often, the bully can't operate alone. There's a little clique or gang with him/her to cheer on the behavior.

Would you join me for a moment to view this from another angle? Let's consider cattle involuntarily "branded", and how we as leaders might wake up one morning and find ourselves "branded" by our corporate communities. Remember Maslow? The need to belong. We do have this need. Do we succumb to our leadership, and like lemmings, do what everyone else is doing? We've been told resilience is the key. Is it? Are you jumping off that same cliff with the lemmings? What's your brand?

Have you ever felt like something evolved in you that challenged your integrity and someone else was responsible for encouraging you to do so?

Could it be because of apathy and/or ambition of yourself or others?

Millions of self-help leadership "how-to" books have been written. I know because I've read many of them and have overflowing bookshelves. In fact, for a good 40 years, it was the only genre I was drawn to read. A slim 200-page or less fast read with graphs, tables, and a juicy business model made for a good recliner curl up for me. My love for these books began with Jim Collins's *Good to Great* classic. It drove my wife crazy as she cuddled with a fat 500+ James Patterson novel the size of a family coffee table Bible! I would read my business nerd books while she would indulge in a crime stopper love epic.

Do you only read for work? Are you curious why? Do you wonder if you're missing something? Have you always said, "I'll read that novel someday when I have time?" Are you reading about your enemy or friend?

This is not a "how to" book with the 27 best steps towards ending bullying. I wanted to write something different from what I have always read to get our attention as a society. In fact, one early critic told me that no one will read this book because of the awkward and missing information and lack of character development. Maybe that person is correct. Guess what? My inner bully agrees, lol.

Kindergarten to the C-Suite

All my life, I've had trials and tribulations. That doesn't make me any more special than the next human. The Bible tells us in the book of James that these trials are ordained to perfect us, and that we may be lacking nothing at the end of our lives. God's ultimate intention is for us to be *resurrected* with Christ, and not just stay the same resilient self. Contrarily, we are called to die to self. There are things we should be strong in the face of. They are the Refiner's fire.

Then there are situations imposed upon us via others' choices or internal lies that we can't understand. If we allow them to continue and internalize, they might destroy us. It's a paradox of life, choices, and hate. How do we know when to be strong and when to refuse it? It's complicated. I don't know the answer. Maybe you do. All I know is I hope to hear "Well done good and faithful servant" someday because of how I adjusted my "one another" mindset and served, rather than sought to be served.

I formed an illusion at a young age that it was expected of me to hold a stiff upper lip and be resilient in the face of bullying. What doesn't kill ya makes ya stronger, right? Jokingly, I feel I may have earned a PhD from the School of Hard Knocks. Bullying is a bad seed and can spread like weeds.

My first experience was in kindergarten, and it was astonishing. My teacher was a young and quite attractive lady. She smiled with pearls of kindness when parents or other teachers were around. When we were alone with her, she duct-taped our mouths shut and plastered posters on the windows so no one could see inside the classroom. It was dark and deafeningly quiet. Every now and then, you would hear a kid whimper because they had to go to the bathroom. A few soiled themselves. It was a prison camp. She did give us paper and crayons so we would take something home to show our parents. Evil, you ask? At lunch, she told us every day, "Children are to be seen and not heard. Eat quietly."

One day, I ran from my parents, away from the bus stop, and crashed into a chain-link fence. Blood was all over my face, and through my desperate tears and snot, I muttered, "I don't want to go to school and be taped."

My dad yelled at me and dragged me into the car. The whole time going to the school he told me I was a bad boy and a liar, and liars go to hell. He said my teacher was a sweet person. My dad even said, "Children are to be seen and not heard. Don't make up hateful stories about people."

Well, the principal, my dad and the teacher were surprised when we showed up mid-morning, unannounced. We discovered an entire kindergarten classroom of taped children and a sleeping teacher who'd left her sleeping pill bottle open on her desk. If I would have continued being resilient in the face of such abuse and said nothing, what would have become of me? How about my classmates? I am not sure. She was arrested and fired. The bullying ceased.

I recall times in middle school when boys put other boys' heads in toilets and called it a "swirly." It was disgusting, and it seemed as though there was an overhead announcement, because everyone knew and pointed or sneered at you if you got one.

I got my share of those.

I liked a girl and wrote her a love note. I attempted to pass it forward on the school bus via my friends that were near her. When she got my note, she turned back, smiling, and motioned for me to come to her seat! I was thrilled, as you can imagine. Once I got there, another girl, a known bully type, grabbed my new girlfriend's hand to steal the note. I intervened by retrieving the torn note. In the furious scramble, the bully clenched her face and teeth, and with rage, her fingernail scratched my right hand between the thumb and forefinger. It bled immediately. I still bear the scar from that experience on my right hand decades later. I tried to do something about a bully I witnessed and got marked for life by it instead. I learned maybe it's best to just let the bully alone, give them what they want and be strong and courageous (Joshua 1:9). Things will return to normal. But they never do.

When I was 8 years old, I was diagnosed with a rare congenital kidney/bladder condition. Four years later, I had major corrective surgery, which landed me in a children's hospital for three months. I had my twelfth birthday there. The doctor who did the surgery hypnotized me and had me imagine my favorite TV show. At that time citizen band (CB) radios were the craze, and my family was really involved in a CB club. I ate, drank, and slept *Moving On*, a series about trucking. (Breaker, breaker One-Niner. This here's the Outlaw-that was my CB handle, "The Outlaw")

My doctor told me and my parents about a miracle he could not explain. He said while I was on the table for several hours having surgery, and because of the successful hypnotism, I only lost a teaspoon of blood! He shined a flashlight in my face and told me to think about my favorite TV show. So, I did.

While I was hypnotized, he said he communicated with me and directed my body to respond. Sounds magical and impossible. Still pretty darn cool, right? The truckers heard of my hospitalization and gave me a ride home from the hospital! I remember when I went back to school, my teacher asked me to share with the class about my experience. I did. The bullies used that information against me and started saying things like, "I'm going to hypnotize you with my fist." Or "Hey, you better 'Move On' before I kick your you-know-what after school." It was relentless and stupid. They just latched on to something I said and used it against me. I don't think I did or said anything to invite it. It just started happening.

I was slammed into lockers, locked in a locker, and pushed out of the showers into the hallways with only a washcloth to cover myself. Yet, I persevered.

KINDERGARTEN TO THE C-SUITE

I was becoming "Mr. Resilience" one insult at a time.

My name is Jim or James. I prefer James. My wife knows and loves me as James. She uses my full name when I'm in trouble! I chose to change it in high school to Vern, my middle name, because I wanted to avoid what became a powerfully widespread name-calling. My parents called me Jamie. There's nothing wrong with the name. It might even be your name. But that became kindling for bully-fueled fires.

There was a popular TV series at that time in my life, *The Bionic Man*, and then the sequel, *Bionic Woman*. Because the woman's name was Jamie, and mine was too, the bullies found the coincidence to be a lot of fun at my expense. They teased and belittled me with name-calling. Sticks and stones may break one's bones, but words sure as hell can hurt you.

I nearly drowned when I was six. I could swim like a fish before that day. Something just happened, and I was underwater for an extended time. It was an accident, but it scared me. I love water to this day, but don't swim. I vividly recall looking through the blue water, seeing the blurred legs and faces of my cousins above me and their muffled voices calling my name. Once I was rescued, I remember the deep coughing as the chlorinated water expelled from my lips and how cold I was.

To graduate high school, it was required to swim the length of the pool. I dreaded that day for four years. I faked an injury or sickness whenever swimming came around in the curriculum for gym class. My fear built a bad reputation for me as a scaredy-cat. I will never forget the far-reaching impact of bullying and name-calling. My horror became real when one teacher learned of my "nickname" and joined the bullies that day. The teacher yelled at me while I was desperately dog paddling to pass the test, "Come on, Jamie! You're the bionic woman. Use your bionics!" Everyone in the pool laughed and pointed, and I sank to the bottom at the end of the pool. I made it. I graduated; but it was truly awful.

I joined the Air Force despite my dad's disagreement, even though he was a Vietnam veteran himself. He refused to sign my enlistment papers. I think because of his experience in Vietnam, he had PTSD and may just have suffered too much. I try to think of it as a form of compassion he had for me by trying to protect me from joining and reliving his life.

I did very well in Basic Military Training and Technical School. There were none of the ghosts of the past to haunt me, only fresh new friends and leaders who wanted to make me into the best airman I could be for my country.

During my first duty assignment, I met a supervisor who said to me, "You are my white boy slave, and you will do whatever I say, Airman. Do you get me, boy?" I thought maybe my dad was right. That guy got demoted, though, and I was moved to a flying squadron, which was a lot of fun. I didn't report him. It just worked out that way for my benefit.

My next boss was an officer who had been passed over a few times for full bird colonel. He was brash, and he didn't like me from the start because my uniform was too crisp. He told me that and wrote me up for being out of uniform. My boss told me weekly that I needed a haircut, too. He was bald, and I had a full head of unruly, thick hair. One day I shaved my head. He wrote me up for looking unnatural in uniform. He wore a flight suit, and he didn't like my Air Force blue uniform. I could never have worn a flight suit.

He just kept needling at everything I did, to the point one day I decided, just like in kindergarten, not to go to school. By noon, the Military Police were knocking on my door, and I was headed to correctional custody for going AWOL. He had me right where he wanted me-out.

A chief master sergeant who knew me stepped in because he was fed up with the bullying officer's behaviors and treatment of me and other airmen. He was strong and strict with me, but because of his intervention and saying something about what he witnessed, the officer was removed from his post and demoted. I graduated non-commissioned officer prep school as the honor graduate, just like the chief said I could. I learned a lot about servanthood from that senior enlisted leader. He saved me and mentored me.

Thereafter, I did well in the USAF, garnering best in the Strategic Air Command in my career field. I only left the service due to strength drawdowns by then President Clinton. Otherwise, I would have stayed. I bled blue with dedication and love of service. I had one more USAF boss that I will refrain from discussing. The impact this narcissistic abuser had on me lasts to this day. The story is embedded in one of the upcoming chapters.

I did a lot of different jobs after the service. I sold used cars, wiped butts, was a therapeutic assistant in a mental health ward, and I was even a special events coordinator for Easter Seals. I had decent bosses and colleagues. I did my job, went home, loved my family, and wanted more success. So, I went to the university and finished a bachelor's and master's in speech pathology in short time. There was only one job in all the UP available – I got it. The company then filed bankruptcy, and I was forced to open my own practice.

The department head for one of my contracts didn't seem to care for my personality, possibly because his staff gravitated towards me. I pulled up outside the school only to see this man rifling through my desk. I approached him and he denied it. He then ended the contract! To this day, I have no idea why. I will say this, his son became one of my good friends and even a student. The man was a good man. He just asserted his power in a way he may have felt at the time was justified. I must have done something that made him uncomfortable. The challenge is, we never, and I mean *never*, got to discuss it.

After I was fired, he asked me to help his son get into the university program where I served as a faculty member. I graciously assisted him and his son with the application, and well, the rest is history. The man has since passed on. It was a confusing time and sequence of events.

At my very first civilian corporate leadership strategic planning summit, we did a team exercise where a member of the executive team was part of our group. The rules of the exercise were clearly laid out that the executives were not to act as leaders, but instead as team members. The game involved assembling a tower together using string, tape, and spaghetti noodles. My team leader was "leading." I reminded the group of the rules, and the leader put the masking tape over my mouth. Everyone nervously laughed because they kind of had to. Talk about déjà vu!

At that same meeting, the group discussed whole health and hypnotism as a strategic new service. The speaker asked if anyone had experiences with hypnotism. I told my childhood story. A physician in the group stood up and called me a liar. He said that it was impossible to lose that small amount of blood. It was quite embarrassing, and it triggered a flashback. I caved inward and spoke no more in that meeting. Despite learning to keep personal details to myself, I always seemed to have something to say and a desire to share my experience with others. I wanted to be part of it and help.

Years later, I was selected for a C-Suite role. I thought to myself, *Now I can make a difference for the better.* A person who also competed for the role but did not get selected came into my new office and said to me, "You know, we both applied for this job." I thought to myself, *Yeah, and I got it.* Frozen in shock, I said nothing. I internalized my thoughts and feelings. Those words stuck with me and did not help my confidence or my suppression of confused anger towards that person. I was dismayed at their gall.

The irony is, my new boss convinced me we would honor the greater good by helping this person. We offered them a temporary assignment in our C-Suite. The hope was it might work out. It didn't. The whole time this individual was on temp duty, they undermined my credibility behind my back with my direct reports, my boss, and with the new executive team that had selected me, not them. Everyone felt it necessary to tell me how my credibility was being challenged by this person in private. No one officially did anything about it. Some of the team believed the lies and distanced themselves from me.

Once that person's term ended, we discovered their failures and poor judgment. I was determined and stood in the way of the important projects to protect my organization. Even then, I was criticized as being a barrier. I never received affirmation. My gut was right. Maybe I was the problem? Still, neither my supervisor nor any of the rest of that team said anything to me. Why, you ask? I wondered why, too!

Things could have turned out quite differently for this person and maybe they would have been invited to our team. Instead, pride and narcissism ruled. We thanked and dismissed the individual at the end of the temporary assignment. What a relief for me, but the months of walking on unnecessary eggshells in my new role created delays in my productivity and trust building. I had to make up for the time lost once the environment became stable. Damage was done. I was not the same and my team had doubts.

There's another nearly final episode in this saga of bullying that I chose. My choice led me to a dark place in my life and career that motivates me to do better. Again, this story may be hidden in future chapters as I recoil at the grotesque and selfish nature of what happened and who it happened to by the hands of a system and bad actors. Heroes were harmed.

I was told by a pastor that he had only heard one negative thing about me as the new CEO. He shared, "People say he's just so happy. Why is he happy all the time?" He even told my wife this. She was perplexed. I wonder if bullies can smell a potential victim. Is there something about joyful, humble, helpful, and dedicated people that invite abuse? Why do we do this to one another? Why do we gang up to support bullies? Should we even call someone a victim? I didn't choose to be one. Did you? Have you chosen to make someone feel victimized?

Normal Reactions to Abnormal Situations

I am not seeking your sympathy or empathy because I know many of you, like me, have been bullied to some extent at some time or witnessed it. You might even think I am some awkward social nerd of sorts and have a serious mental condition-I'm not. You're not. What this is, is a ***normal reaction to an abnormal situation***.

I don't start every day intending to be rude or obnoxious to people. My feet hit the floor every single morning and I say with my left foot "Thank" and with my right foot "You" to God for a new day and then I ask, "What can I do to serve you and others today, Lord?" Have you wondered if some people just have a bully bullseye painted on them from birth while others are designed to be throwing the darts? Is it just that way?

Some of us have bullied others, and believe it or not, that's a sort of normal outcome. Everyone wants their way and looks out for number one, versus someone else's betterment at some point when the stakes are high enough. I am not judging you, and please don't judge me. My hope is through this book and by cultivating your curiosity, you better understand and choose to change yourself and your world.

We all need to. Here's the science why:

> *People die from stress. Bullying antagonizes our organizational, individual, and societal health. Our paucity of intentional awareness and presence fosters subtle internal physical and mental stressors that, over time, erode relationships and peace.*

> *One might say:*

> *What you permit, you promote.*

When God Shows Up to Coach Mr. Resilience

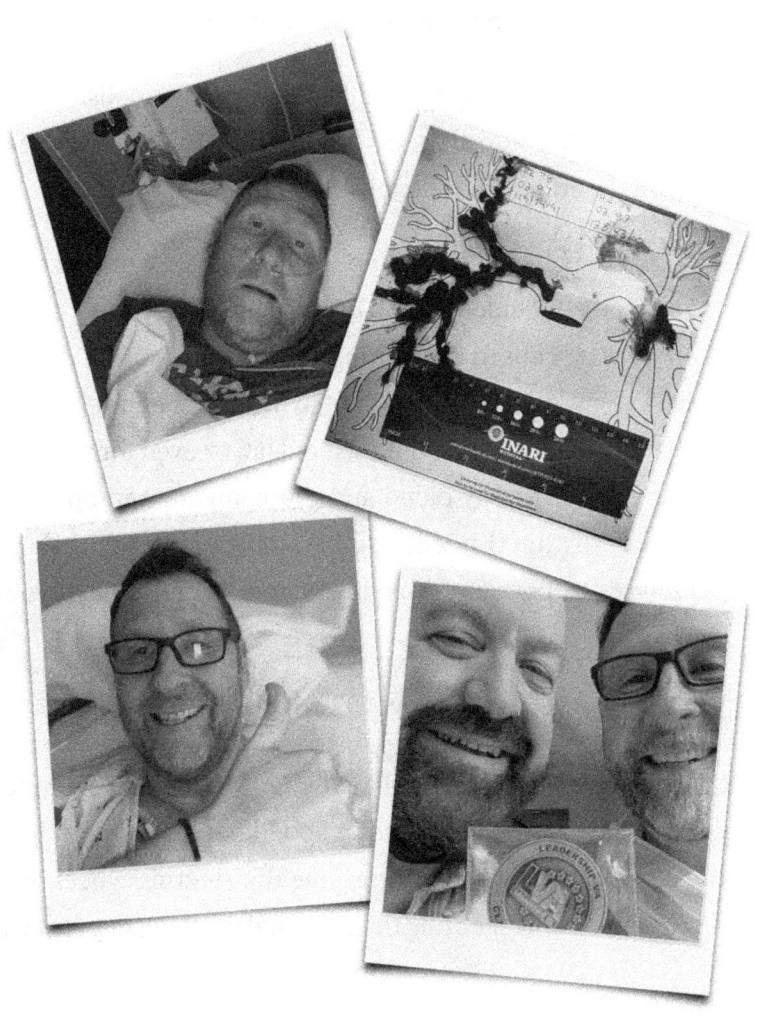

The sequence of pictures you see here are:

1. Selfie of me in the ICU.

2. The Autopsy Plate holding hundreds of clots removed from my lungs.

3. Me post-surgery.

4. Me "coining" my doctor who saved my life.

I had a massive saddle-type double pulmonary embolism. This is the picture the doc shared with my wife mid-surgery. No words can describe what she must have thought.

He and his team ruled out all possibilities of its cause except for *stress*. This included COVID or vaccination. Nope, it was *chronic stress*, caused by putting up with too much drama and pressure at work. Too much bullying, too much tolerating people acting badly-saying things about, at, or even for me. Too little life/work/harmony blend and too many misappropriated priorities of my life. I needed to be awakened to life. I share these images to perhaps awaken you and prevent this in your life.

Here's my story:

On Christmas Eve, 2022, I collided with Mr. Resilience. I met my life/career choices. I was not a good life passenger. In fact, I was crawling over the seat, grasping the steering wheel, and trying to drive while ignoring the signs and crashing into myself.

WHEN GOD SHOWS UP TO COACH MR. RESILIENCE

What unfolded that night was remarkable. It challenged my core and faith. From about 11PM until 1AM, I felt and heard a strong presence in my bedroom. I will refer to the presence as an angel. It said to me either audibly or in my spirt, "Stay awake. Stay with me. Call the hospital." Being a stubborn man, I wrestled with this presence, just like Jacob did. I felt something physical pushing me off my right side to my left and we wrestled back and forth for hours. It was odd, yet I could really feel something pushing me over. Thankfully, this angel did not break my hip! I gave in and called the hospital. The triage nurse listened intently to my symptoms of shortness of breath and sharp pain whenever I turned on my right side.

My wife was sleeping in the guest room. She had caringly given me space for some peaceful rest. The triage nurse insisted I put my phone on speaker and go wake my wife. She yelled my wife's name to get her to the phone as I stumbled down the hallway to wake her. The nurse told my wife I was having a pulmonary embolism or suffering cardiac arrest, and we needed to hang up and dial 911. To make a long story short, we called 911.

An ambulance came, and the paramedics tested me, stating, "Nothing is wrong with you." Now we were facing a substantial medical transportation bill. Because of VA rules, I had to go to the hospital or else pay a big bill. I told the doctor my story, and he believed me. He was a Christian. On Christmas Eve, he called in a full interventional radiology and CT staff before really knowing what was going on with me. After seven hours of tests and waiting, he told me, "You have minutes to live due to a double pulmonary embolism and there are hundreds of clots in your leg, hip, and lungs, as well as a severe pressure against the right side of your heart. We must move fast."

The top item on my to-do list that day became: Just breathe.

> *That was my wake-up call from God that I wasn't Mr. Resilience.*

I decided to put my family and *self-care before healthcare*, which had been my career path for four decades.

> *I mistakenly made it my life path, likely to prove something to myself and others about me and my implicit bias, based on experiences to live up to my self-identity as Mr. Resilience.*

I'm no famous person, minister, or leader; however, the primary focus of this book is not about me. Although, I've shared a lot. Maybe even TMI! My intent is to provide you with emotionally evoking fictional stories about the various types of bullying that should pique your curiosity. The goal is to explore your life journey and how it makes you "show up."

Despite being given a life-or-death notice, I lost sight and took another C-Suite Role-CEO. I hadn't learned a thing. I thought Mr. Resilience could still persevere. Well, Mr. Resilience walked out of that C-Suite without saying goodbye. Lots of reasons, mostly mine.

One thing is for certain... none of us can truly plan our path.

See the Church See the Steeple...

My grandmother used to say, "The perfect church is one with no people. The best church is one with a lot of different ones."

We want to be safe. We want food and shelter. We want to belong.

Our grandmothers would not be too impressed seeing we let our culture degrade into name-calling and a tsunami of selfish bullying that rules our life and workplace. It erodes psychological safety and threatens us with commonplace mass shootings.

Violence and distrust are everyday events in our lives. It's almost as unremarkable as radio static. As humans, we continue seeking to honor or forget the historic COVID-19 pandemic and its scandal. The lies, mystery, coverup or truth may never be known. Mixing this cancerous cacophony together in a big bowl, the recipe yields a world ripe for bullying. It comes in all shapes and sizes, both internalized and externally imposed. The good news is: ***We still have a choice.***

The choice to bully arises among peers, subordinates, or superiors, and even loved ones. It can be experienced in any direction: laterally, downward, and upward. It's a human thing, and like any church, if it were void of people, would we still possibly bully ourselves with self-defeating messages? I think of the adage, "If a tree fell in a forest and there was no one around to hear it, would it still make noise?"

In my professional field of healthcare, an unexpected bully arose in 2020-2021-COVID-19. We were forced to wear masks in public places for years and were dissociated from families and friends. All our meetings were on our computer screen monitors. We barely got up from our desks to go see someone. It was, and still is, a stressful era to live in. This post-COVID tsunami brought interesting dimensions to life and work for us all. The uncertain nature of our trust evaporated between leaders and those they led. Even families were divided. We met a new bully, the cyber-bully. Because we couldn't get in the same room physically, we resorted to using emojis and words. Our churches became perfect and empty.

Healthcare saw unprecedented, rapid, unexpected departures of C-suite leaders. Doctors, nurses, therapists, and ancillary staff have also felt the pangs of post-COVID life/work decisions. Burnout became a reality. These were proven and good people who worked hard to arrive in life and career, actualizing their "people-helping" abilities at the highest organizational levels. I counted myself as one of them. In some circles, we call it a calling or servant leadership.

During the pandemic, uncertainty of information caused leaders to fail, with no real chance of succeeding. Leadership requires information to make wise decisions, but the information kept changing. Thus, the direction from leadership felt like a constant state of confusion and anxiety. The pandemic created a tumult of toxic, confused or scared people making accusations, organizations failing to support the leader, or burnout. Let's not forget the media and politics. Ugh. These elements drove good people to persist in the name of *resilience*. As you may have guessed, I thrived in that environment because it gave me the opportunity to really show how tough I was.

Why? Because we were taught to. It makes you a better leader and more respected when you are seen as resilient and get results.

Some just walked out or were pushed away to other pursuits, including early retirement.

Somewhere along the way, this word *resilience* became vogue, and no longer just associated with material properties. It became a human accomplishment. Leaders resorted to reassuring one another that being *resilient* is how we fight the good fight. We say it's for the greater good. By being tough and resilient, you will return stronger. Now wait a minute! Stronger? That is not congruent with returning to our normal shape and/or function. It's improved: smarter, stronger, better looking, and more hair! We heard this all too often. It's like its own gospel now.

If you do an internet search for the word resilience, you will find countless books, seminars, articles, memes, you name it, that glorify this word/concept into something of a savior for the professional person to strive towards. What is true is we have come to accept that bully behavior is included and is to be silently tolerated to just get things done and be inclusive, respecting everyone.

World leaders call each other names as if they were in the fourth grade. In church, we learned about a guy named Solomon. He was the wisest. Remember what he said in Ecclesiastes, "...there is nothing new under the sun." It's all vanity. Well, our leaders are acting like fourth grade bullies. They isolate characteristics or a short momentary lapse in someone's political, military, or family history to defame them. Again, it's to get the big "W". Yet clouded by media, supporting them is the only answer for our countries and world betterment. We cautiously laugh as we become bystanders to this WWE of world-stage bullying. Ask yourself if you or a friend haven't repeated the banter to support of your own beliefs. This, my friend, is the heart of bullying.

We have great hesitation now to honor "see something—say something—do something". Only when the evidence is so powerfully present and lawfully indisputable will we take any action now. The litigious nature of *leading with fear* has paralyzed us. When we should be screaming from the mountain tops, "Stop the madness!", we sit dormant in the name of tolerance. Does it even matter? Will anything ever change? Often, the perpetrators are promoted or allowed to fade into another form of existence elsewhere. In a game of hockey, the offender is not the one sent to the penalty box; the "retaliator" is. Who wronged whom? Be sure that a leopard does not change its spots, and the grass isn't greener. The leopard we call *resilience* does sound super cool and might serve as an exhortation to some. Truthfully, it boils down to *playing and working while injured*. We continue to grasp false hope it will heal alone and return us to our normal shape and function. Humans can't do that.

That is an illusion and a lie.

The long-range impact of being resilient to bullying changes people's lives.

We can, however, influence our environment through intentional and regular awareness and action. Moldy bread is moldy because it was left out too long. Again, what you permit, you promote.

Crooked Road Ahead

Stories: How to Read this Book

Have you ever been driving and seen those wonderful yellow diamond-shaped signs: Slippery When Wet, Animal Crossing, Falling Rock, etc.? Your attention is guided to a different or dangerous condition to keep you safe and alert. My writing style is intentional. You may become uncomfortable with it at times. Warning: **awkward and shifty content ahead**. Why? Confusion. It manifests in your brain and body chemistry, leading to reacting or freezing. You might even throw the book!

Think about how you feel, where you feel, and when you're taken by surprise in a real challenge or bullying experience. It's our pre-flight simulator. You know that feeling in your gut when something isn't right, true, honest, lovely, transparent, complete, or lawful? Or worse yet, you regret your own actions, or you are made to feel small? Give yourself permission to have this inner talk while reading. Be mindful to compare your experience. Envision how you might leverage your patience and kindness response if you were in the place of a character. Aim for understanding toward self and others. Be super curious and non-judgmental.

It's easy to read juicy stories of other people's plight without immersing ourselves, not in the story, but in the self-discovery experience. Our stories form an "implicit bias." Be aware of what that is for you. This is why I told you some sordid details about my life. I certainly have a clouded lens too; but it's my lens. You have yours.

To the elephant in the room: I refrained from the potential of missing out on honoring our differences. I choose to address difference and diversity as a real aspect of bullying in this manner: I ascribe, we are created equal. If any characters are of a diverse background, etc.... those are referred to as "purple polka-dotted" to give awareness only. We know this form of bullying or discrimination exists historically and even still today, sadly. There may have been a better way, but to preserve anonymity of the brave contributors, I'll use "purple polka-dotted."

I find it compelling that the Bible has over 1,200 verses with the words "one another." To set spiritual value relative to a chapter, I've added those for your meditation. We collect pearls of wisdom from the people who influence us. There's a "pearl" too for your consideration.

Remember, when you're frustrated or confused, this is by intent to stimulate your emotion and open your imagination wide.

Presence Pause

I did not foresee myself in an interventional radiology suite on Christmas Eve, fighting for my life-*but it happened*.

I also didn't see myself ignoring that signal-*but I did*.

I didn't see I was losing touch with the ones I loved most-*but I was*.

I didn't see that the guy looking back at me in the mirror wasn't my authentic self-*but I should have*.

Finally, I didn't see my unplanned, abrupt retirement and leaving the public service I so loved-healthcare for veterans like me.

But I had to.

I realized I needed a Presence Pause for myself. I realized it needed to be intentional and easy to use. I also saw a vision of resurrection and a new me, no longer Mr. Resilient's return.

I changed. My mindset changed.

Here, my goal is to share insights, navigating the changing landscape of leadership and the illusive "executive presence." Can we call it "presence" for the purpose of this read? *Presence* and *being* are a good *prevent defense* to raise our awareness of bullying in ourselves and one another. For centuries, mystics have told us to meditate. We grab our super caffeine-charged latte and head to the gym or a mountaintop to do yoga. It might just be a little easier than that, my friends.

When was the last time you looked at a tree, a ladybug, a rock, a window with beveled glass, a blade of grass, a child at play, a roadway or bridge, or anything for that matter, and really studied it curiously for a few moments, thinking of nothing else? Reading is a live, interactive form of meditation when you are present. **When we read for work and continued education, we are still at work! Think about it.**

I believe being present in life is the answer. Don't just let life pass by. *BE* in it. We can't effectively learn without intentional focus. In conversation, we can hear and not listen; but we cannot listen without hearing. In reading, it is best when we interact and are provided specific space to just notice. Please read somewhere quiet and ensure you have dedicated time. Think, and try to feel each story.

Listen carefully to yourself. Watch your body, your thoughts, and your emotions.

You will find "**PRESENCE PAUSE**" strategically ends each chapter. Please stop and notice yourself using the SCAN2WIN method described below. They look like this:

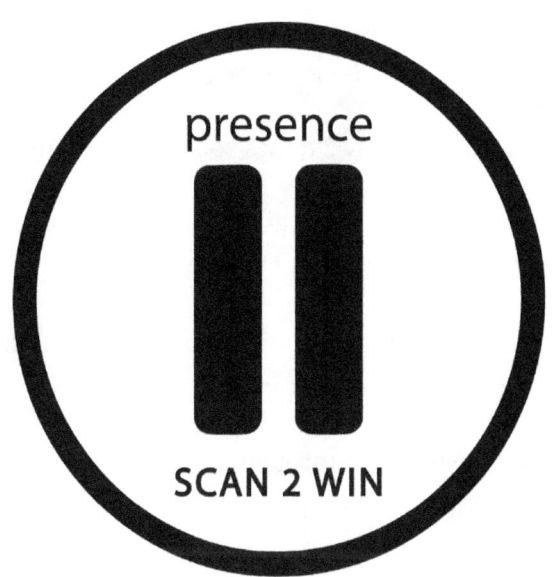

PRESENCE PAUSE:

SCAN2WIN: **S**ense, **C**uriosity, **A**lign, **N**ame, **2** (To), **W**in, **I**ntegrate, **N**avigate

Here's how each component fits:

- **S**ense: Begin by sensing your physical and emotional responses in the moment.

- **C**uriosity: Cultivate curiosity about what's triggering your emotions and reactions.

- **A**lign: Assess how your reactions align with your core values and biases.

- **N**ame: Name and identify your emotions to understand them better. Name behaviors.

- **2**: Take time to say 2 things you are grateful for out loud.

- **W**in: Focus on strategies and actions to effectively handle the situation and "win" the day.

- **I**ntegrate: Integrate your insights and understanding into your response strategy.

- **N**avigate: Navigate through the situation with clarity and composure, applying what you've learned.

SCAN2WIN provides a structured approach to self-awareness and emotional management, aiming to help you handle challenging situations effectively and maintain control.

Some Science to Ponder

Hang with me for a second, while I get a little deep and nerdy about this. Stress fosters increased chemical levels of cortisol. Higher cortisol levels trigger our body's immune response, which results in inflammation that can be anywhere in our body and brain. If the injury or condition is perpetuated in a chronic pattern, it becomes a serious health risk. For instance, we can be scared to our core when we see a wolf pouncing towards us with teeth gleaming. In this situation, the heightened cortisol level and our response leaves us three options: We can freeze, flee, or take the wolf head-on in self-defense. We also might see that same wolf from a safe distance and cautiously, but calmly, admire its beauty while considering our prevent-defense, should it become necessary.

Please use each **PRESENCE PAUSE** as an intentional measure of the physical and mental changes you notice in yourself while reading each story in this book. The variety of situations and people types are specifically written *to get to you*. To ping up against your *values*. To make you *curious*.

Why should we simulate getting stressed by reading a book about a stressful topic? So together, we can better understand our stimulus and response patterns that push us to ***lead with*** *fear*. This is not courageous leadership or life. It is reactive and can be impulsive and painful for the leader and those following or living with you.

Leading or living with fear is a barrier to finding our authentic self and achieving an effective executive presence.

Leading and living with fear keeps some of us from addressing or calling out situations or people. In the Bible, this is encouraged as spurring one another toward good deeds.

For a meta view, let's say that wolf is a substance abuse issue in someone's life. Let's consider alcohol consumption. One can drink responsibly. Well, some can. Isn't it ironic that we sometimes go to get a drink after work? We even call it "Happy Hour." Sometimes, we NEED a drink after work. Some have said coyly, "This is why we drink at our desks." When something goes awry or is overwhelming at work or home or both, you've probably heard something akin and laughed along with the sarcasm.

The truth of the matter is that substances increase our cortisol levels. Did you know that? When our cortisol levels are elevated, guess what we typically do? We become afraid, angry, sad, depressed, overjoyed, super excitable, or exhausted. Regardless of the impact, it's because of the increased cortisol in our bodies. It has been estimated that after having a drinking episode, it can take a week during the withdrawal period to return to normal cortisol levels and maybe never. Are you

SOME SCIENCE TO PONDER 43

tracking where I'm going with this little science/biology lesson? Here's a fun equation to consider:

If cortisol is stress, and alcohol consumption increases cortisol, the simple math equation disproves our illusion that a drink after work is a stress reliever! It worsens our condition.

Some "happy" hour.

Drinking during work would not be highly recommended either.

Neurologists have long known and advised persons who have succumbed to traumatic brain injury or stroke to abstain from alcohol entirely, as it is like pouring gasoline on a fire and ends the lives of many neurons. When we can't think or speak, we become fearful and stressed. Then where do we go? To our primitive brain stem and long-term memories (implicit bias). This is where we try to ensure our root desire to survive and be the fittest or last one standing. Our working memory and short-term memory are experiencing a neurological power outage and are unavailable to us to help us reason. This is a danger zone. It doesn't always take alcohol or other substances.

Here's another wolf to consider. Are you an adrenaline junkie? Is it under control? Have you experienced the withdrawal and similar conditions of a substance abuser? You might say I'm stepping on toes here, and that discussing going fast, having fun on a motorcycle, or jumping out of a perfectly sound aircraft is judgmental. Bear with me. Adrenaline seeking, substance abuse, and bullying have something in common: Exercising those activities/behaviors results in a conditioned, higher threshold of tolerance. The challenge is: the more you do, the more you need; the more you need to be in control, the more you control; the more adverse your activities, the more you increase the adversity or risk to get the rush.

Could this be why bullying is so repetitive and some spectators join in? Could this be why so many young athletes and celebrities find themselves as the cause of a fatal situation or accident, from their reckless choices to feed the adrenaline wolf? Is it love of the fight for the sake of the fight? Are we married to rules or committed to our principles and values? Do we have to make our own rules and force others to follow them just because we made them? Are you curious what you might find if you could mount a cortisol level meter on your desk? Would it be revealing to you and those around you? Believe it or not, it can be done with a saliva sample... or a simple PRESENCE PAUSE!

> **Children and adults who bully others have been noted to have *lower cortisol levels* because their threshold for stress is higher than those whom they target. They enjoy, and are rewarded with, chemical courage; and like any other addictive behavior, they need more to get the same high.**

Call to Action!

Wouldn't it be wonderful if reading this book resulted in one less human suffering at the hands of a bully-namely you?

Let's do this for *one another*.

These stories are genuine experiences; bullying of real people who shared anonymously. No contributor would send me an email. Every human wanted to just chat with me, to protect themselves and others. That is how powerful bullying is. There is no age, race, ethnicity, etc.—***nothing exempts any human*** from this experience. It's real. It's visceral. It's mean-spirited. It can be boisterous or silent. It must stop.

> *Bullying lingers for years, decades, and perhaps generations.*

You may find what I am about to say controversial, but give it some cognitive space. Bullying sprouts from who you are or who you want to be, and worse yet, who others try to tell you that you are. By being ourselves, we can be perceived as a bully. When we apply our strengths and gifts, considering one another with care, we can contribute positively and be productive as team and life mates. But if we sense, recognize, accentuate and/or strive to *one-up another and act or think upon it,* bullying becomes chronically unhealthy.

Here's how we can further recognize bullying:

Ask yourself these powerful questions:

1) At times, <u>do I sense</u> what will challenge, belittle, or trigger another's identity, beliefs, fears, confidence, guilt, or other life experiences?

2) At times, <u>do I recognize</u> traits/characteristics in others to exploit them and gain an upper hand in relationships?

3) At times, <u>do I accentuate</u> myself over another?

4) At times, <u>do I strive</u> to be the Relationship Power Broker?

Don't judge how you answered. Instead, reward yourself for being brave enough to honestly do so. We now have a start!

The power of bullying can be exacerbated by concomitant conditions. Our gifts are especially powerful, debilitating, and may be deadly if the bully or bullied person also has moral injury, traumatic brain or physical injury, and/or chronic stress. We can't know everything about everyone. Some people don't want others to know.

We must just assume that our choices and actions impact others.

You really can't make this stuff up!

CALL TO ACTION!

Life happens, and people collide.

Can we watch for warning signs and drive safer?

I will draw upon my own life and career experience in the military, higher education, healthcare and as an appointed Senior Executive Service (SES) with the Veterans Health Administration (VA). Because of my military and VA background, I added highlights in some of the stories. Additionally, you'll find some touches of culture and language common to Michigan's Upper Peninsula. My wife and I raised our family there, and I encourage you to consider visiting. In the fall, the leaves changing color is nothing short of spectacular. You'll find ice sculptures the size of buildings in the winter. In the summer, there are the majestic Great Lakes, especially Lake Superior. I love the white fish! You must try a Lawry's pasty (a meat, potato, and vegetable pie). Trust me.

I will offer one answer that I am certain of. A lady asked me an intuitive question after reading one of the stories you are about to experience. She asked, "Do all bullies know they are bullies?" While I was writing this book, a person from my past commented on a social media post of mine related to bullying and this book. The person wrote a lengthy proclamation that I had bullied them in a meeting. This was a public forum. Well, as you can see from the very first words of the book, my confession: I am a bully. So that takes the sting out of the discrediting defamation attempt, for me at least. I reported the post. How could this person ever know what I've gone through in my life? Maybe the only answer in this book I am willing to commit to is:

"No, all bullies are not aware, and I will add from my research, not everyone knows what bullying is."

Perhaps a good follow up question we could explore together is:

"Who, what, where, when and how does my inner bully manifest?"

A last and very important disclaimer: It is my *aim* that we are okay with the fact there is a bully in one another and can move forward. Our gifts, implicit biases, or choices can in any given situation, and with any audience, "show up" like the Incredible Hulk or a vampire sucking the life out of a room or person. OR they can be beautiful and helpful. Does the costume fit?

This is our presence. This is our executive presence.

Now, let's appreciate what many of us call derailers. I'm curious. Maybe there's another way to look at this. Rather than derailers, could this simply be understood as an *architecture of choices* which facilitate or disrupt relationships? We do have a choice to seek truth and reality, dropping our illusions of each other. Does the train have to be derailed?

I've adopted three key terms to watch for. Below is my foundational definition:

Injured Reserve: *A sports metaphor. When we allow chronic stress or situations to persist, absent of healing and we keep on keeping on. We continue to pursue daily, or stay in the game of* life, love, work, or play while we should be paying attention to the signals of health. Injuries can be physical or emotional.

Integrity Revealed: *The quality of having a strong moral compass and a relentless refusal to compromise, while being fully honest with self and others. Our integrity is revealed when recognizable by self or others that we place care in our choices and actions. In contrast, lack of integrity can be revealed when one makes an opposite decision to avoid or ignore integrity.*

Chronic Stress: *Stress leads to heart, lung, and immune conditions, which can be seriously exacerbated if noticed, yet not addressed. Stress can be acute, or chronic and cyclic. Our bodies answer this via our immune system. By continuing to address a wound that won't heal, the body becomes inflamed. This inflammation can be just about anywhere, including our brains. Once activated and producing chemical healing agents, it is not easily shut off when we have chronic and continued stress. These neurological conditions can, and have, contributed to people taking their own lives.* ***It can be deadly.***

The next Entity is Insight. Remember, these are real events for the most part. Honor confidentiality, even if you think you or someone you know may have contributed. It's not about the contributor. It's about the contribution!

ENTITY TWO
INSIGHTS

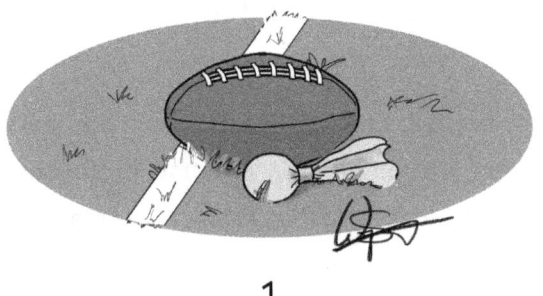

1

Minister of Defense - Injured Reserve List

Ephesians 4:32 "Be kind to one another."

Pearl: "Principles always win over rules when it comes to doing the right thing."

Have you heard of the "Minister of Defense?" Not the political type, but a sports figure? Two-time National Defensive End, ordained minister, and National Football League great, Reginald (Reggie) Howard White, of the Philadelphia Eagles, Green Bay Packers, and Carolina Panthers. He lived and played for years while on the *injured reserve (IR)* list, yet achieved greatness and a Super Bowl XXXI win. The injured reserve (IR) is supposed to represent a holding place for players who cannot or should not play in a game until healed. Reggie became known as the "Minister of Defense", not of his own acclaim, but by his teammates.

At a very young age, he is reported to have told his mother all he wanted to be when he grew up was a professional football player and a minister. At 17, Mr. White was ordained and had a successful school sports career. In 1982, he found himself on the IR, but was able to get 47 tackles and was named the team's top rusher. He could have easily made the NFL, but instead chose to continue to refine his ability in the United States Football League.

During a game, an opponent cut blocked him and caused an injury. Cut block is when a defensive player hits an offensive player from behind, below the knees. It can be a career-ending dirty play. White lined up the next play and asked his opposer if he knew Jesus!

In 1985, Reggie became Rookie of the Year for the Philadelphia Eagles. The Eagles didn't do so well, but Reggie did. Buddy Ryan, who was a defensively minded leader, became Reggie's mentor and head coach. Under his mentorship, the Eagles improved alongside Reggie, and his *integrity was revealed*. White's numbers continued to improve, but in 1992 tragedy struck as his friend and linemate, Jerome Brown, and a family member were killed in an auto accident. Losing this friend impacted Mr. White significantly.

The Eagles finally made the playoffs but without further advancement, and Reggie was ready for a new challenge, so he set out as a free agent. Reggie and others found themselves labeled as rebels and faced a lawsuit posed by the NFL to prevent this. Believe it or not, the owner of the Eagles reportedly bullied Reggie and his family during the negotiation period in a passive-aggressive manner, to the point lawyers and agents got involved. He allegedly said to Reggie when he was requesting reasonable and equal pay something to the effect, "...you're a Christian. You shouldn't be worried about money so much." Talk about hitting to one's core. NFL rules highly discouraged free agency at the time, but Reggie was able to do it with God's calling, his gift of influence, and an angel negotiator named Ray Rhoades, the Green Bay Packers' defensive coordinator. During an interview, Reggie was asked how he would know what team to go with and he replied, "I will listen to God. He will tell me where to go." But the funny thing was that the Packers' head coach, Mike Holmgren, called Reggie and allegedly said, "This is God. Come to Green Bay!"

Principles always win over rules when it comes to doing the right thing.

The move to the cold country of Wisconsin was not without challenge or politics. The Packers and the Green Bay area were sparse with African American people's presence. That area was also referred to as "Siberia, where no good player goes." So, there was that! Still, Reggie heard God's calling and answered despite other lucrative options. Because Reggie took the path God laid before him, which was indeed the "one less taken", he was able to recruit top-level teammates, who just happened to be African American men. They won the Super Bowl.

Remember the cut block I mentioned earlier in Reggie's career? It happened again against the Dallas Cowboys, when a friend and fierce competitor, Mike Williams, cut block Reggie in a divisional game the Packers lost. It placed Reggie on the IR, but a miracle happened... Reggie was healed and able to play in the next game! Reggie had an amazing career as a Packer. Read his book. It is well worth it.

Sadly, in 1998, White abruptly retired, sending shockwaves through his organization and the Green Bay community because his *integrity* had brought him great favor in a place where it did not previously exist. He built that favor with man because he had favor with God and chose to represent doing the right thing. A year later, he re-joined the NFL with the Carolina Panthers.

White's retirement was not without more politics. As a minister, he had his beliefs, and his expression of those beliefs led to his falling out of favor with the rich and powerful, resulting in a loss of sponsorship and money. Then, as suddenly as his first retirement, he passed away on December 26, 2004, at the early age of 43. His life and career were cut short by a disease—cardiac and pulmonary sarcoidosis, which affected his sleep and cardiac-respiratory health. White's ministry, leadership and path touched so many lives. His generosity was endless, and he was renown as a servant and friend of God.

It was in the 1980s when my family visited a church in Midland, MI, where we first met Mr. White. The next day we went to a Chucky Cheese, and wow, there he was, real and towering in height and his overall size. He was a giant man.

MINISTER OF DEFENSE – INJURED RESERVE LIST

Do you know what he did? He *revealed his integrity*. He was humbly dressed, and there with his own family for an afternoon together. Despite having a busy life in which he had limited family time, he spared a precious moment to speak with our children, as if they were his own. He left them with words of encouragement to "Keep going to church and *be kind to others*." That moment still resonates with our kids. When he passed, it was as if we had lost a family member, too. There's humor in life and sports—we are Detroit Lions fans!

There are great and egregious rivalries between sports fans. The NFC North is a notorious home for this fun. At times, disturbing inter-relationships with the people who root for "their" team develop. Vicarious bullying is a real thing. Sometimes it goes a bit too far. It becomes an if-this-then-that concept.

Let me expand. Because you are a fan of a team, you now are associated with them, their winning or losing record, and as such, you are a winner or a loser. It's like the Dr. Seuss book, "The Sneetches." There are those with stars on their bellies (in-crowd, fortunate, cool kids) and those without (outcast, losers, less fortunate, nerds, etc.). There have been fights and even shootings at games. There have been massive celebrations and dark depression from loss. The effort that goes into sports is enormous. This effort and striving goes back to gladiator times. Remember what happened then? Somebody always got killed or eaten by a lion.

How many times during a game are you texting or talking trash? Is it fun, sarcastic, or mean-spirited? Do you find hate rising in you or them because someone shared statistics of a team that has been "rebuilding since the 1950s"? Or pointing to past failures of the new coach like he was on the 0-16 team now that he's a coach? Stuff like that can be fun or can be furious and frivolous.

Last year, my Lions made it to the next-to-last game of the NFC Championship and fell short. Fans from other teams, especially one, felt it necessary to poke and prod even though their team was not in that game. Of course, their team had been there many times before and holds a beautiful time-tested legacy. Not this year, buddy. The fact is, our inner bullies love sports because we can blame or hide behind our teams and not ourselves.

Some really identify with sports based on their implicit bias and life experiences. I've been a Lions fan since my childhood. Yeah, they lose a ton of times. Yeah, they struggle. Yeah, they're from my home state. You can pick your nose, but sometimes you can't pick your battles because they are picked for you by an arm-chair quarterback or washed-out high-school athlete, or just someone who likes to get a rise out of someone else. At any rate, isn't it a blast having nachos, chicken wings and friends to enjoy a game wearing your favorite jersey?

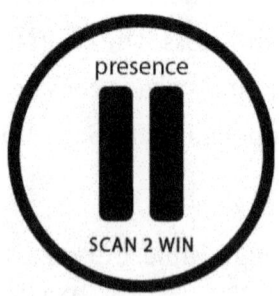

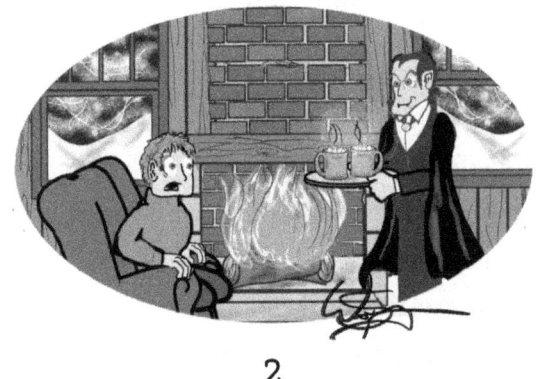

2

Snowed in with Dracula

Ezekiel and Sage

Philippians 2:4 "Be interested in one another."

Pearl: "Did you want five words or my advice?"

Ezekiel

My wife Miriam and I were on a ski vacation in northern Nevada at the acclaimed Lake Tahoe. It was still nearly 80 at our Florida home, but we longed for the beauty and majesty of snow. It was a beautiful lodge, and several hundred guests were huddled in because of a major winter storm. The snow was pristine and looked like white diamonds in the reflection of the lodge's flood lamps; yet it was coming too fast, preventing the groomers from keeping up, so the hills were closed.

While sipping our coffee, we started up the normal small talk with an older couple, Sage and Sarah, from Georgia. Right away Sage and his wife sounded like the movie *Deliverance* with that intriguing and adorable southern drawl! I found it delicious to my ears. He asked what I did, and I said I was a hospital CEO with Riper. He exclaimed, "I did 'time' with Riper Healthcare Systems (RHS) and several others over my 48 years!" I had just finished my probation year, and he was an experienced leader, but coincidentally, we were both healthcare CEOs. Small world, indeed.

As the conversation went on, our wives both gasped simultaneously at our "work talk" and took off to some boutique. He and I laughed, clinked coffee cups, and got right back to the topics of the weather and work. We both groaned about the current storm. He really caught me off guard when out of nowhere my new acquaintance switched his thick southern accent and started channeling a stranger, "Fer sure, it's like da Jack Frost, Mitter Freede and Dracula are runnin' da weder, dontcha know!"

At first, I had no idea what was happening or what to say, then we both laughed our butts off. I said, "Was that a bad scene from the movie *Fargo*?"

He explained, "No, that was my terrible impression of a Yooper friend of mine!" He continued, "Yeah, a friend of mine, who was also a healthcare CEO with the famous RHS, just like you." He said those words and, I guess, as odd as they are, they stuck with me. Well, more the way he said them as he described the weather in the Upper Peninsula of Michigan where he was from.

I said, "That's an original statement. Unique and oddly appropriate for what's going on outside now."

Sage

Yes, I will never forget that guy. He had a lot of unique ways of saying things. He claimed he got them from mentors, but some were quite off-the-cuff and often flipped backwards. I am convinced he made them up as he went. He was a personality of his making and history. He was a good leader and a heck of a teacher and storyteller, but he could be tough to understand at times if his accent or language differences were too colorfully Yooper. I guess our southernisms can get Sarah and me in trouble at times with certain folk.

It could have been that he knocked his noggin a couple of times badly while in the military. I have heard that people with traumatic brain injury history, like many veterans, have similar challenges. Jazz served in the Air Force.

Ezekiel

Sage asked me if I was a veteran.

I replied, "Yes, sir. 25 years Army, I made it to colonel. In fact, my whole family, back to the Civil War, served. Well, my dad was a three-star general in the Marines. I didn't get to his level. He was tough on me. I tried but couldn't stay in to be a general. Too much death and dying, and I have a love for food, so my waistline failed inspection often. As a kid, I never belonged anywhere. We were always on the move because of my dad's career. We also have a nephew who was a Marine, who is now a federal lawyer. I joined healthcare as my way of giving back."

Sage

That is quite the rich history! Sarah and I have our home in Georgia Peach country still. Jazz convinced us about Michigan. So, we have a summer cottage on Lake Huron. It's a little place called Oscoda. They say it was where Paul Bunyan was born. It is where we go to get away.

Jazz retired about a year or so after I did. It was quite abrupt. He just got up and walked away from his first CEO job ever. I picked him for the position because I have hired tons of CEOs. I told him I'd been watching him for a couple of years and it was his path. I even went a step further and told him I was pretty sure God agreed. He said that mattered very much to him in his decision to take the position.

When I asked why he had to leave RHS and healthcare, Jazz told me he had played on the "injured reserve" list too long. The toxicity was just too much. He had his share of bad bosses before me and a few investigations. He once told me that one of his underlings refused to do something because they didn't understand his speech. Then that employee filed an EEO against him for discrimination and profiling. He'd had enough.

Ezekiel

Sage said, "Sounds like you two have a bit in common?"

I retorted, "I never quit anything. I retired."

Sage quickly realized the awkward moment I created. He pivoted, saying, "Not easy. Not easy at all."

We agreed that these CEO, or any executive jobs, aren't easy, nor friendly positions nowadays. It seems like everyone is right and has rights except for the leaders. Anyone can say just about anything or complain you're being unfair or mean, and they sit you in a corner with a crayon for months while they investigate you. Worst case, some are handed a cardboard shoe box to vacate. All because some employees and their unions feel they were wronged by being asked for accountability, performance or conduct-related questions as part of being one's supervisor.

I quietly pondered how on earth someone with a TBI history could survive such rigor of being a CEO, too? I thought of the good people I knew that left jobs because of stress, drama, trauma, and bad players. I thought of the soldiers we lost in the Army. I thought of the families and those damned envelopes.

My inner voice hit me, *My God, I'm dealing with shenanigans at the hands of passive-aggressive bullies and self-centered people. All the while, I'm trying to drive our healthcare in the best direction for patients. Sometimes it feels like the leaders are just waiting me out to move on to the next thing. Seems like a lot of my time is spent dealing with personnel and interpersonal or communication breakdowns versus commitment and strategy.*

It was like I heard Miriam chastising me from afar for talking about work and getting myself spun up. I stopped my inner pity party and asked my new acquaintance, "Sir, if you had five words to share with a new CEO, what would they be?"

He smiled in a devious sort of way and said, "Well... show up, be real, be you, be nice, keep commitments."

I said, "Well... that's ten words in five pairs."

He seemed to not like my quipped attempt at humor. He retorted, "That's what I am talking about! Did you want 5 words or my advice?"

Sage had hit my bullseye.

Sage

You see, we as leaders fear we need to be the expert. That's wrong. We think if we are, then no one can pull the woolly blanket over us. What we need to be are the cheerleaders and visionaries. This is what is discouraging a bunch of long-term leaders into retirement, like me. We can't lead; we wind up being fear mongers. We think everything is ours, so we must be the only one to fix it. Again, not true! That's unnecessary pressure we put on ourselves. We're too busy worrying about rules and deathly afraid of letting anyone inside our identity or emotions to know us authentically. It's somewhat because of the risk of our litigious healthcare and unionized environments that we walk on eggshells and miss the mark. If we told someone our truth, they'd likely use it against us somehow. It's endless. We must navigate a minefield all day, every day. God forbid, we bend a little to do what principle is right, versus what rule is written. So, to save our hides, we become something they (whoever they are) want us to be. A lot of times it's not corporate or accreditation bodies. It's the people we work with and for us. Sometimes our own families. Culture is a complex dynamic and can be hostile long-term due to the players involved and our total disregard for one another.

Ezekiel

I thought to myself, *Man, I thought I was jaded!*

Sage waxed melancholy. "Jazz was himself; he knew how to show up and he didn't mince words with people. It was about patient safety and care for him and me. I guess that's what I saw in him. I also want to see the best in all people. Sarah lovingly calls me an old fool. But I know it's a blind spot, and it cost me. Of course, there are those few parading about who claim to have values, yet are surreptitiously striving for their Lexus, fancy suits, and titles. Damn narcissists!"

We clinked our cups in honor and memory of the good people; but I added to our toast, "There are few nobler callings than healthcare! To those for their service and resilience to fight while wounded!".

"Resilience—I don't know about that," said Sage. We both felt disdain for the word resilience and wondered why anyone would want to be resilient in the face of bullying.

Sage went on, "Jazz lives in the UP on some back road far from everything and everyone. I still hear from him infrequently and I touch base too. It's been a while."

Sage asked me if I wanted to hear a defining story in Jazz's life. I said, "Well, pour me another coffee and maybe we'll add some Jameson to keep things going. I would like to know why Dracula was in his weather report!"

He laughed. "That was Jazz's drink of choice, straight up on a few rocks!"

He began channeling a bad version of the Bob and Doug McKenzie show "Up North" with ... "and Jazz said" the respectful impersonation began:

Sage began, "Static and da broke signal was all dat would dial in dere on my liddle Radio Shack AM/FM. Ever now's and denz, dat announcer's voice would break tru da static. 'Awful. Worst in years. Tens of inches of snow, black ice, and high, forceful winds with twenty additional inches of wet, heavy snow expected; making driving hazardous over da next two days, dontcha know. God's country, da UP, but da weder is run by Mitter Freede, Dracula, and Ole Man Winter!'"

He returned to his own narration. "Just to let you in on something about Jazz and me, we both hate snow and cold. He would say, 'It's pretty and all dat, but man, she's back-breaking work.'"

Sage showed me pictures of a huge, modified sheet metal shovel with a wide handle, which, according to Jazz, was known as a Yooper Scooper. "We do not have those in peach country yet, but it might be a choice for me as a retirement business niche at our Oscoda cottage! We've never seen winter in Michigan and for good reason. Those Yoopers invented squeegees to push snow off cars and roofs! Hundreds of inches each year."

As Sage continued describing this apocalyptic winter wonderland filled with hearty Finnish women and long, ice-filled bearded men, I felt a chill, even though the fireplace was toasty nearby.

I wondered if Sage and Jazz were related. He sure made an impression on this old man. I squeezed a peek at my watch.

"Jazz shared with me that after his military service, he was in another terrible auto accident when he worked for RHS. It was caused by the weather and black ice."

Talk about luck! I finally got a word in edgewise. "I have had a lot of friends seriously hurt or lost their lives because of the impact wintry weather has on travel and safety." We both agreed that weather, leadership, and military service have a bit in common. They are unpredictable and can be life changing.

I took another secret nod at my watch and said, "Well... since it is going to snow into oblivion," (I channeled my best Yooper)

"We'd best hunker down dere, dontcha know, and find our better halves."

He rolled off his stool, roaring, and complimented me on my attempt, concluding with a fist pump. "Dracula! Dracula, because he sucks like winter weather does, I suppose! Bad pun."

I thanked him for the story, laughs, advice, and Jameson and I found Miriam in the boutique at the register, armed with a new purse, coat, and ski boots!

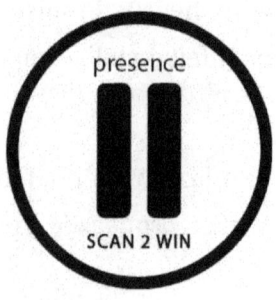

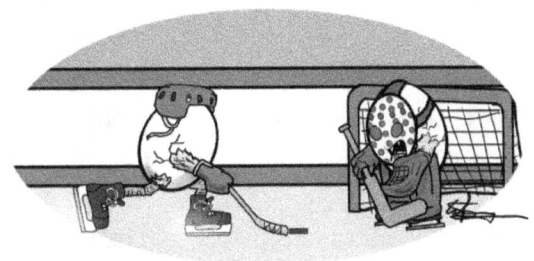

3

Scrambled Chicken Embryos on Ice

Ezekiel and Ryder

Proverbs 15:13 "A glad heart makes a happy face; a broken heart crushes the spirit."

Pearl: "Visible leadership can be seen. That same visibility can become a target."

Ezekiel

My family and I traveled from our southern Ohio home to our son, Abel's junior hockey Midwest Regional Playoff game in north Wisconsin. We enjoyed nachos, brats with sauerkraut, and frosty Leinenkugel's in the translucent plastic cups provided.

What a unique cuisine, but it was tasty! The lady at the concession stand said, "Don't throw these on the ice!"

I texted Sage a pic and told him about the old school hockey town. He texted back: "I bet the Hanson Brothers had played there!"

Wisconsin and Ohio had a strong rivalry. The rink was in a cold, old northern pole barn. There were holes in the barn's wooden walls you could literally see through. The ice was dimly lit, hard and fast. Junior hockey is not glamorous, and it smells of sweat and old socks. The players are in their late teens and honestly, are men trying to make it to the next level. Many of them are taller than 6' and weigh 200 pounds.

Abel was not tall, but was quick, agile, and good in the corners. The team our son was up against were state champions the previous year. They were well known for rough, unruly play on the ice, especially one defenseman named Bubba. No, you can't make a name like that up. Our team was ahead by a goal and there were only a few seconds of the third period remaining, when Abel found himself on a speedy breakaway toward their net. If he buried the puck, our team would have solidified a big win.

The crowd was all standing and pointing at the net. It was exhilarating and horrible all at once, as nachos, brats, and beers went airborne from the shock on our side of the rink. Bubba intercepted Abel from behind as we watched things turned into slow motion. Abel was catapulted past the net into the solid boards from Bubba's desperate and illegal cross check from behind. The place went silent except for the ref's whistle and the crowd's collective gasp.

Bubba's mother exclaimed, "Way to go, Bubba!" from across the ice. Her screechy voice stirred an unholy anger deep within me. More importantly, I ran down the bleachers and awkwardly shuffled like Tim Conway across the ice with the team's new athletic trainer holding my hand, even though I had never met him.

Abel was piled up like a bunch of laundry, not moving. I had a PTSD moment, fearing the worst had happened to my son. My gut was tight, and tears welled up behind my eyes that I, as a good soldier, held back. I could hear the old general criticizing my feeling of vulnerability. The trainer slid to his side and sat on his butt on the ice. He didn't kneel and *oddly, I noticed that*.

He began his assessment as Abel slowly rose to the clamorous roar of relief from the crowd. Either I imagined it, or the guy mumbled something like, "Why do these tragedies keep happening around me?" The trainer recommended we get a CT scan to ensure there was no concussion or brain bleed.

One last obligatory face-off, the clock expired, and the buzzer blasted, signaling the end of the game and our bittersweet victory. Helmets and gloves were in the air as we quickly navigated off the ice and out of the arena.

When we arrived in the parking lot, we were interrupted by Bubba's mother, an equally intimidating woman. Bubba didn't fall far from that apple tree! She accused us of teaching our son to skate wrong and cheating to win.

I thought, *Now ain't that something? Accusing us of the very thing she is guilty of.* I sometimes have anger bursts from my military experiences, and I verbally let loose on her about raising a bully. I shared a few choice words as I described her and her hit-man son as "pieces of poop". Miriam pushed me into our minivan, and we rushed off to the nearby hospital.

The athletic trainer met us there. Once in the hospital, he and I had a moment to talk. He got right down to business, and we didn't even introduce ourselves to one another. The trainer was all business, no bedside manner. He described concussions and their aftermath. He said we needed to do neuro checks on our son, as it was a bad hit from behind. "Helmets are good, but they don't guard against the contra coup (brain movement in opposite direction from the point of impact)." He drew a quick picture of the brain and points of impact. I noticed his dirty fingernails. Black like oil or gardening. I nodded and kept my infection quality control thoughts to myself.

We then started up some small talk. He sounded familiar to me. We discovered he was stationed at Eielson AFB, Alaska, and I was at Fort Wainwright Army Base as an Army air traffic controller. He explained how he knew so much about these types of head injuries, as he was in the Air Force and had a runway accident in the 80s.

I abruptly stopped him and said, "Hey wait a minute? Are you Ryder? The driver of that ole Big Blue?" "Yeah, that's me!" the trainer enthusiastically responded. We instinctively hugged. I told him I was the ATC that night and was so glad he was okay. We then began reminiscing together, reliving that terrible early Alaskan morning.

Ryder started. "It was like any other exercise except it was bitter cold and our shift ended after midnight. I just remember us grunting, cussing, sounds of tugging and our laughter echoing through the thick, frozen, still Alaskan air. It was 0200 AM. Jazz, my dorm mate and I were doffing our cold-weather gear."

I thought to myself, *Jazz? How many of those are out there?*

Ryder

Jazz complained, "Four days of wearing this costume!" He always had me in stitches. Jazz had a funny way with words. He tried to lighten my mood by pretending to be a documentary host describing our uniform as we changed at the end of the shift. He did weird stuff like that all the time. I just got used to it. He was my friend.

Jazz started this odd, but hilarious, commentary. I remember it like it was yesterday because *it was right before it happened*: Bunny Boots. They were named that because, when inflated, they appear like a snowshoe rabbit's foot—more like Mickey Mouse! The higher ups say these boots can keep an airman's feet warm in temperatures as low as −60 degrees, yet you navigate like a 1-year-old, and the snow squeaks so loud under them you could not hear an elephant sneaking up. Great military equipment!

Now these Bunny Pants look nothing like a rabbit, but they do make you look like a contestant on the Richard Simmons show. They are awkward, held up by suspenders that constantly slip and lose their grip. So, while standing guard under a B-52, you are constantly pulling up your trousers and readjusting your balls like a baseball player stepping in and out of the batter's box.

Then there is the parka! Another cruel invention of military fashion designers attempting to copy an indigenous Inuit's glamourous fur-lined and soft parka, which was typically made of fine mink and polar bear hides. Ha! Not even close! The military-issue parka is more like they used tent canvas and plywood and lined the hood with needles taken from the back side of a white porcupine! It is neither soft nor elegant, and tastes horrible because you inhale the white hairs when the hood is closed and fully zipped, leaving only a three-inch round hole to see out. So, there you stand, looking like a sitting duck in drab green with a furry white beak.

Folks, here's the finale—the mitten. The mitten measures three feet in length and is covered with what appears to be the butt of a bison! I was bawling and laughing but gathered my military bearing because I outranked him by a stripe, and I bellowed an order out, "Get in the truck, you Yooper!"

Ezekiel

Ryder and I shared a good belly laugh after that story. I knew there were two in the truck. I just didn't know the other airman. I also wasn't ready to break Sage's confidentiality.

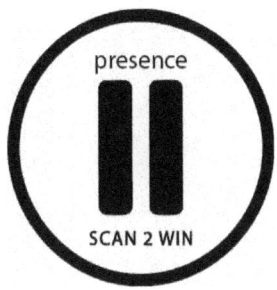

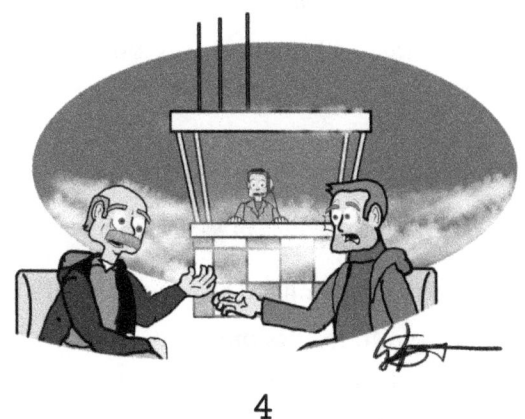

4

Coming Clean

Ryder and Ezekiel

James 5:16 "Confess to one another."

Pearl: "Tell the truth, the whole truth, and clarify."

Ezekiel

"I recognized your voice, man," I told Ryder. "I remember the exchange that night was like any other exercise. I did my job."

We began reenacting the whole dialogue like it was a good military memory. "Tower to Mobile Security Two, otherwise known as 'Big Blue'. Clear on northbound A4 for crossing at the two-miler mark, over."

Ryder added, "Roger that, tower. Visibility limited to a few feet. Ice fog is thick and reflective. Tarmac is greased with ice. The last temperature was −43 degrees. Big blue two affirmative, over."

"I remember teasing you, too, as we always do. Army vs. Air Force," I told Ryder.

"Affirmative for cross two-miler. Have a good night, gentlemen. It's been a long, cold four days out here. Ya done good for Air Force. I know you wingnut boys are headed to your fancy chow hall for some fresh scrambled chicken embryos and pigskins! We have MREs (Meals Ready to Eat) here. Typical Army!"

Then I covered the potential hazards left on the runway. "Only traffic is home and parked: a C-5 Galaxy Cargo, that old BUFF, and not much else visual or planned. They're both on A5 so you boys are clear." I thought, *What a night for the ground control team to call off. I got a lot to pay attention to here now.*

~Author's Note: The C-5 Galaxy is the largest cargo aircraft. Very hard to miss that beast. Its full load capacity is just over 281,000 pounds. Semis fit inside it. The B-52 Stratofortress Bomber was named by pilots as a BUFF, aka Big Ugly Fat Fellow. The B-52 could potentially be armed with nuclear weaponry. To maintain national security, none of us could either confirm or deny the presence of such weapons. MREs were disgusting, but highly nourishing fare issued to the military in case we couldn't get to a proper dining facility. ~

"When you boys gonna get a new truck? Over."

"Your truck sure stuck out among our Army green," I told Ryder.

"It was fugly," he acknowledged. Ryder continued, "I remember it well, man. It haunts me as it was the beginning of the end of our great friendship, oddly."

I sensed there was an underlying message yet to be told about that as Ryder continued, and I was glad I hadn't mentioned meeting Sage, who maybe knew Ryder's partner Jazz. The awkwardness started to rise. I remember what happened, just not the final outcome.

Ryder

Jazz was in the passenger seat of "Big Blue", our canvas-covered security Chevy crew cab K30 pickup. Ya know, we named it like pilots do their planes. Don't you guys name tanks? We caught all kinds of flack for using that as our call sign.

Jazz was my dorm roommate and friend, as well as a heck of a guitar player. Jazz always wanted to be Randy Rhoades from Ozzy, and I wanted to be Rudy Sarzo, as I play bass. He sure played well, and he wrote the song that got us on a sweet musical tour. He was a religion freak. I stayed away from churches and hypocrites. Anyway, we had our dreams of rocking a coliseum someday, but then we did make the Alaskan Air Command Talent Travel Team together.

Ezekiel

I congratulated him on that, hoping this story wasn't going where I was sensing. I could almost feel my feet slipping from under me, but they were still there. I could see them.

Ryder got back on track about the incident. "I was driving and responsible. We had been out on security post for four days to support the joint forces extreme cold weather exercise with you guys at Army Fort Wainwright."

I tried to redirect him. "It was a big deal. Even some squadrons from the lower 48, including Nellis AFB, Las Vegas, were participants." I added, "I remember we had several flyovers from across the pond (Russia) during that one, which made it exciting for us in the tower."

Ryder

Exciting! That was unnerving! We were exhausted and glad the exercise was over. Your voice was reassuring and gave us our path out of danger. Thanks for that. Jazz and I talked about it during radio silence. "I wonder if that was an exercise, eh?" he asked me. "What ya mean, man?" I remember Jazz mentioned the constant strafing of the MiGs *(Russian fighter aircraft)* and our F-16s lighting up the after burners *(F-16 US Fighter Aircraft)!* Those were some chases! There was a lot of action. Kept me warm, sort of. It didn't seem like an exercise to me. At times, my heart was pounding like Neil Pert's double kick bass drum. I thought we were goners.

I was an aircraft fuels maintenance man by classification back then. I liked to think of myself as tough. I grew up in the inner city, and, well, you had to be tough. I was a bit more war-savvy, and typically had greasy, blackened hands and fingernails, and I smelled of JP4 *(Aircraft jelled fuel)*. I was an Air Force grunt. Jazz, on the other hand, "pushed a pencil and flew a desk", as we say in the USAF to describe office or support personnel. I lovingly called him an ivory tower pansy.

I remember telling Jazz, "Happens all the time, man." It was especially busy this time. I kidded him that HQ (Headquarters) called up the Kremlin, and they had side bets on who could chase who first! He scared a lot easier than I did, and I felt like a big brother to the guy.

I distinctly recall my last words to Jazz: "Nothing to worry about, man. Let's get some chow!"

Ezekiel

I thought, *Last words... oh no, here we go.*

Ryder leaned forward into my personal space, and his voice lowered into the ire of the moment. "In that split second, our world dropped into an awkward precision and pace like that of a KC-135 Tanker and C-5 Galaxy refueling, as I had described to Jazz so many times—it's deafeningly slow."

Then Ryder really got to the gory details.

Ryder

I don't sleep much. Sometimes I have terrible headaches, and I can see it like it just happened. The horrible sequence that night began with Jazz screaming, "SWAT!" My whole body instantly froze, yet I was able to move somehow. I hit the brakes; the black ice was as unforgiving as an Olympic luge run. While Big Blue skidded, the Peacekeeper SWAT beast came into clear view out the passenger side window, headed right at us with no break in speed. It was so odd, because I could see Jazz's side of his head and the Peacekeeper's headlights jamming towards us at the speed of an Iron Maiden lick.

~Author's note: Peacekeepers are huge, known as the Cadillac Gage Ranger, and the predecessor of the modern Humvee. They were often used as a SWAT (Special Weapons and Tactics Team). It's an armored security vehicle weighing around 10,000 pounds when fully loaded, and they can hit 70 mph, although a typical runway speed limit is 15 mph.~

Ezekiel

Ryder's voice raised, and his forehead tightened down on his bushy eyebrows. "But that night, man, some Army team was joy riding, and the military police estimated the speed of impact was 50 mph!"

There it was...

There was this awkward silence between us because right then, I could not speak. My heart sank, and I knew I needed to excuse myself to go puke, but my feet had suddenly slipped from under me. Was Ryder processing this while I was punishing myself, getting ready for the onslaught? He changed his posture and sat back, uncrossed his arms and legs, and slowed his breathing. It was like he was doing it on purpose or something. It was as if the world froze for me while my inner bully beat on me and formulated excuses—I was the ATC in the tower. I had no idea those idiots were on the runway; it all had happened so fast. I was left alone, no backup. No one watching the ground. The tower team was at discord with one another. A couple of the ATC guys, not me, well maybe me, were tough on the ground crew. Some name calling and maybe someone took a bunch of batteries out of truck radios to get them in trouble during this exercise. I knew that.

It got ugly. One guy was so angered he took a swing at an ATC. ATCs are officers. Ground is enlisted. Fights were not highly looked upon. The stupid bullying and back and forth at the dorms and at the job started to impact our mission readiness. The ATC reported it and the whole ground team was on mandatory kitchen duty.

I told Ryder they were safe. I felt like I was about to be slammed into the boards by my past mistakes, of all places, at a hockey game, and Ryder was my Bubba.

Ryder remained peaceful and quiet. I still tried to cover up and spoke softly and slowly. "Ryder, being an ATC is not a profession for the light-hearted and neither is healthcare administration, which I am in now. In the military, we pride ourselves on precision and safety as paramount." In my mind the echo was, that night I owned their demise, or at least deep in the dark parts of my memory banks, I did. I had been on shift too long. Somebody else could have filled in. I was responsible overall. I wondered if Ryder could hear the voices. He saw my smokescreen, I'm sure.

As the proverbial referee's whistle blew, I got up off the ice, and I could physically hear Ryder again. Ryder didn't cross check me. I ran into the boards myself. Ryder continued with some profound words I'll never forget, because from my raised vantage point in the tower, it all happened so quickly. It was like a matchbox car accident, and it was because we failed as a team to get along.

Ryder

If Hell has a sound of fury, it was replicated in the wee morning hours on January 7, 1983, the coldest day that year. I remember hearing Jazz scream, "Jesus!". All the glass in Big Blue spontaneously disintegrated into microscopic shards. The impact seemed about as slow and painful as an immunization needle piercing the skin and then the burn. The sound of crinkling metal was met with the nose of that evil SWAT penetrating the passenger door.

Jazz was pinned immediately. I could see his right knee was crushed. I could see the Army driver's face as he braced for the full impact. I remember going forward and hitting the glass, but thank goodness, not exiting. The sheer driving force was like a bulldozer relentlessly shoving us as Big Blue took to the air flying, swirling, and rolling to a final resting spot, upside down on its cab roof.

I couldn't do anything to protect my friend or myself. We were told it was a quarter mile from the point of impact where we stopped. During these hideous gyrations, Jazz and I looked like a couple of astronauts defying gravity and both of us hit our heads multiple times on the side and roof of Big Blue. Once the commotion had ended, I imagine there was the typical eerie silence, then steam hissing, spinning wheels, sirens, whirring of the SWAT's engine—as if it were a bully proud of its psychological warfare, flashing lights and voices. Lots of voices. There was also a saw sound of grinding through the metal roof. I guess that was to extract the two of us from the mangle.

I remember my right leg being very warm and mushy feeling. Somehow, I didn't fly out of Big Blue. The doctors thought I would have been better off and asked me why I was not wearing full cold weather gear like my bunny pants. They thought the proper gear might have prevented my leg from being exposed when I slid downward. By regulation, we were supposed to stay in uniform until back at our squadron. They surmised that my direct weight broke the gear shift. I sort of remember rubbing my blurry and glass-filled eyes. I have nightmares and I see lots of blood and my leg fully penetrated by the gear shifter. There was shiny metal going in and shiny metal coming out. I was stuck there. I think that might have been when I passed out.

I limp now.

Strange; however, neither Jazz nor I heard or remembered much of it. Yet, for some weird reason, it's in my subconscious and nightmares to this day. We were told we were unconscious and bleeding. I do remember there was glass everywhere and all over me.

Once freed by the firefighters, we were rushed by ambulance to the nearby Eielson AFB Hospital and then quickly moved to Fort Wainwright. CT scans and a myriad of other tests were performed. Guess what the military hospital said in our medical records? "Motor vehicle accident, driver at fault for driving too fast for conditions, two souls aboard a large pickup truck." Final diagnoses were written as, "Some contusions and mild concussion, mild loss of consciousness up to four minutes, resolved at time of discharge. Treatment plan: three days' sick leave. Follow up with primary care as needed. Case referred to respective squadron commanders for disposition." I got bullied by the system.

As we were wheeled out to the bus, a nurse stopped us and gave us both challenge coins. They had a saying on them, "Put on the Full Armor of God." I've carried that ever since, but I keep my distance from churches. I believe in God. I just think he doesn't like me much.

(Yeah Dad, thanks for the beatings.)

It was like nothing bad happened, according to the doctors. We were sent back to work. Jazz to his plush office and me back to the grimy flight line. It felt like no one cared. Well, I guess they were right, because all I really remember was being sore for a couple months and having a lot of headaches.

On top of that, I got kicked out of the Air Force. We didn't make chow, but we did get scrambled like eggs.

Ezekiel

I couldn't believe Ryder's disposition to crack a joke after all that. I still held my disclosure like a fart in church.

Ryder

I went to school to become an athletic trainer and help people with concussions because I know them well. Believe it or not, the Air Force dishonorably discharged me under Article 15 based on that medical record entry. I wasn't even at fault. The SWAT hit us!

Jazz and I were never the same. We quickly grew apart; probably because we were both so angry and short-tempered with one another. We just couldn't gel anymore, and he blamed me that his rhythm on guitar was horrible after the accident. He went on in the Air Force. We never spoke again. It sucked because I had to struggle through school on my own. No GI Bill for me. No disability pay or service connection either.

In aircraft maintenance, we have a saying about our dirty fingernails and smelly uniforms: "Grime and grit makes air power zoom." Well, I got grit, and my life has been smeared with some grime. The headaches, light sensitivity, anger, depression all still exist, but I do my best. I have my own garage where I still do mechanic work. I'm growing into this athletics gig. Someday, I might have clean hands.

Ezekiel

I felt such an overwhelming guilt. My hands were twice as dirty as Ryder's greasy fingernails. It must have been painted on my face, because then something glorious and unexpected happened. Ryder asked me, "Man, you okay? You look white as a ghost."

It was like he hadn't made the cognitive connection or chose not to. I was that ATC somehow, even though we just rehearsed the whole thing. I had to tell him, so I confessed clearly. "Ryder, I was working on no sleep. I was a bull-headed, results-driven kind of Army officer trying to impress. I should have gotten help. There are rules, like you said. I should have been court-martialed, too. My whole team should have been. We were a mess. Fighting and bullying each other. Ground didn't have radios because of us. They got us back by calling off sick that night so we would be short-handed. I always wondered why the Peacekeeper crew was only reprimanded and stayed in service."

Now I know Ryder was scapegoated.

I told Ryder, "When I was interviewed by the military police and my boss, my own *integrity* failed me. I told them we had radio technical difficulties, and that I did tell the Air Force driver about the Peacekeepers on duty and to be cautious. I LIED, man, to save my hide, and ground's, for not showing up."

Ryder pushed back a bit and looked me squarely in the eye. It was awful. I just knew he was going to tell me off in ten languages. I deserved it. This was my deserved cross-check from behind. Brace yourself, Zeke, he's coming.

Instead, this fine airman, who was wrongfully discharged and whose path had led him to helping Abel, said, "Sir, it was my honor to serve alongside you. Your honesty here today and this weird fateful injury has restored faith in me that there is a God and He is watching over us and your boy. You're a good dad. Wish mine was like half of you. I always carried a chip on my shoulder. I despised the tower for not telling us and wondered if any of you knew or what. How could something like that happen? Ice fog is horrible stuff, and I could barely see. We were crawling, and I felt safe with your direction, so we proceeded. Did our job too."

Ryder continued. "I totally forgive you, even though you don't need to be forgiven. You should not regret your actions for my benefit. War is war and very unpredictable, even if it is an exercise. We were playing it like for real it was war. Integrity is a funny thing, and I know it haunts you, too. Wow, did you ever think this would happen? Us meeting like this!"

I could not believe it and didn't need a CT scan. I felt exonerated by his grace, like all the gaps were filled in for both of us. Except that one—Jazz and Sage.

Just then, the doctor emerged with Abel. She dropped the news, just like Ryder said. It wasn't good, but not too bad either. We needed to do neuro checks hourly due to an obvious concussion syndrome. She gave us some strong morphine and sent us on our way.

Ryder and I hugged and exchanged phone numbers. My wife had just come into the waiting room from the van. She looked quite puzzled as I hugged our unknown new athletic trainer and not our son. We got in our van, and I assured her I would explain what happened. I did say this, "Son, that was a close one. We're so blessed you're going to be okay. Honey, it was an amazing connection and a remarkable episode of forgiveness. Too much to go into now. Let's go home."

Abel exclaimed from the back seat as the morphine was kicking in, "Hey, do I get a victory pizza or what?!"

My wife reached over to touch my hand and asked me if I had my wallet. I reached for my jacket pocket and there was Ryder's precious challenge coin!

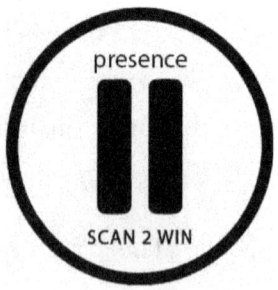

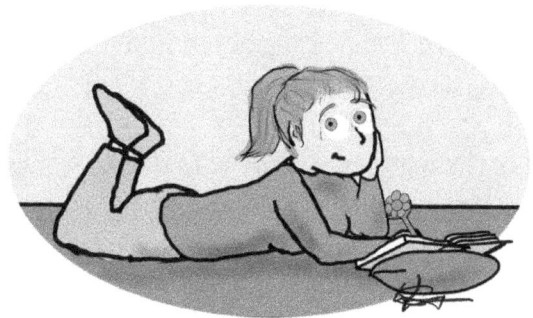

Belle's Diary: Entry One

Dear Diary, Today was the wedding reception. I am excited for them. Someday, maybe me. Anyway, we piled on the city bus, all six of us college girls in dresses, and off to the National Guard Armory we went. The smell of diesel—yuck! I felt hot and somewhat nauseous and really, the mood of being at a reception was fading for me.

Once we got there, the snow was falling hard and getting windy. Another Upper Peninsula storm was brewing. My friends were excited because there was a live band. I just wanted to polka some and have some yummy wedding cake!

Well, Dear Diary, as the night went on, my friend was talking with band members on break, and she dragged one of them over to our table, right up to me! I told her I was simply aghast at the outfit one of them was wearing: a spiked dog collar and pleather black shiny pants. He did have a nice smile and hair, but honestly, this is the UP, not Hollywood. He was shy but talkative. There was something about him, but I didn't know what it was—maybe a special kindness.

At the end of the night, he asked me to dance. No way. Lots of pressure from my friends. "He's cute. He's a wing nut." We all exclaimed out loud in unison, "He's got a car and a job!"

Many Yooper college girls just want their MRS degree, but not me. I have dreams, so that is not my goal. I was okay meeting him, (not really), this gent with a jazzy name, Jazz. Hmmm....

Well, now it is 1100AM the next day and he just left my apartment. Not what you're thinking, Dear Diary. My friend gave him my address, and he showed up at like 3 in the morning, still in that ridiculous getup and wanting to "talk."

Of course, the storm had really kicked in and he mentioned not wanting to drive all the way back to the Air Force Base. So, we chatted for hours on my front entry inside stairs and then wound up at Big Boy for a buffet breakfast. It was nice. I agreed to a second time to do something. He pulled away in his parent's station wagon. Hmmm....

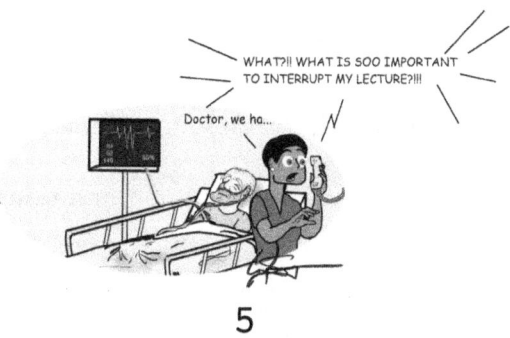

5

Purple Polka-Dotted - Back to School

Ruth and Luke

Ephesians 5:21 "Be accountable to one another."

Pearl: "Trust, but verify and verify again."

Luke

I was deep in thought at my desk when the abrupt buzzing of my vibrating cellphone just about slid it off my desk. There was no caller ID. I found that odd, and possibly spam-related, but picked up and answered. "Luke here. Who is this, please?"

There was a dead silence, and I thought for sure it was a prank or telemarketer of some sort. Then I heard the soft sound of sobbing, and she said, "It's me, Ruth."

I asked, "Ruth, are you okay? You sound distraught."

She replied, "Luke, I am terrible. I am under investigation, temporarily removed out of my position. I feel like a criminal, yet I've done nothing wrong but hold people accountable."

I knew something was up when Ruth called me Luke. I admit it. I've lived a silver spoon life and, yeah, I went to both Harvard and Yale. I'm an MBA and physician turned CEO. She knows I like my toys. We're a lot alike, so we hit it off. She teased me and called me "Harvey Yale." I must keep my distance from her as sometimes I sense she might be a bit sweet on me. My wife would tar and feather me. She didn't bother with the flirting or fun today.

Ruth's voice was shaky as she whispered, "I'm so glad you picked up. I bought one of those pay-as-you-go cell phones that can't be tracked. Remember when we spoke about my new role here and how I am supposed to be 'cleaning house'? Well, it's a long story. Do you have time? I could use a friend."

"Absolutely. What's on your heart and mind?" I thought, *Why does everyone call me when they're having problems? Okay, that was selfish. Focus Luke.*

Ruth gained her composure and began unfolding her tale:

"The team here brought me concerns regarding our access to care challenges. One of my most trusted staff showed me we had a lot of doctors, like 64 or so, that she was sure were not properly credentialed or privileged at our hospital. She assured me she was working on it."

I believed her. She's sharp.

"About a week after the discovery, an interesting situation in our emergency department (ED) happened. There was a male patient who came in by ambulance that was under the care of our top radiation oncologist. You know, one of those special unicorns—high priced like you, Harvey Yale. Seems like it would be totally innocent standard ops, right? Not even! Regrettably, the gentleman passed away in our operating room later that afternoon."

I could sense Ruth was still herself, but struggling with the slight bit of flirting.

Ruth

I had no idea how high the levels of pompousness could go. This doctor was on the list of the 64 my staff were recredentialing—making it a bit more complicated. She requested my chief medical officer (CMO) and I co-sign an email to all of them to add some urgency. We did. She had only heard from a handful of docs.

At any rate, the ED Nurse in charge was told by our ED doc that she needed a stat consult with radiation oncology because the patient was well-known, according to his chart. She expressed grave concern for the patient in the ED suite. He was circling the drain. So, the nurse called oncology, and the clerk said, "Doctor X is at the university teaching, and I will not disturb him. He does not like that." The nurse knew the doc well, too. She had some run-ins with him. She said she didn't want to but knew the man's life was in the balance. She contacted the university and finally got to the doc. He picked up the phone and allegedly, per the note given to me, said, "I'm teaching. What do you want that is so important?"

The clerk was, of course, intimidated, and then unbelievably, the bully doc just hung up the phone. Okay, that's bad enough, right?

Well, gets worse and much deeper and darker. My Quality Management Executive Leader (QM) brought another report to me that was anonymously laid on his desk. It came from the ED, as that's what the sticky note had scribbled on it. It alleged that docs were using personal/sick time off (PTO/STO) as "in lieu of" and documenting that they were working on Saturdays for Mondays. I guess that's okay if you're not rescheduling or canceling, impacting our already struggling patient access metrics.

So, we checked it, and sure enough, nearly 90% of the docs not privileged or credentialed properly were also using what is called "in lieu of" in an interesting pattern. The call to the doc was on a Monday at about 1100 AM. His PTO status was "off", and he worked in lieu of the previous Saturday. Some *integrity*, huh? He was double dipping at the university while his patient

PURPLE POLKA-DOTTED – BACK TO SCHOOL

was dying. He is also part of a group of docs that have revolted against our CMO by filing a harassment complaint. I had to tell my CMO she had to take the call. None of these docs are on call until the complaint is completed.

Anyway, that's not why I am under investigation. It is just crazy how this is evolving. No one is saying that the doc's unavailability contributed to an already very ill patient's demise, but it didn't help, considering the circumstances.

We contacted Human Resources (HR), and they recommended a review and offered to assist. Their first step was to pull the doc from clinical work. Where do you put a doc like that? We decided the electronic records team could use a subject matter expert. Seemed like a good fit.

While this was being processed, I felt it necessary to reach out to the university dean of medicine and compare notes on the accountability and safety between our two organizations. I brought some key team members with me. You know I'm a "purple polka-dotted" person. I am also type-A all the way, like you. I burned the candle and put together a comprehensive briefing paper to guide our discussion. It could become quite formal, depending upon everyone's perspectives and willingness to address. It was quite surprising, but a senator was sitting right next to the dean. She made a point to mention she was an alumnus. I told them about the potential for double dipping and our failure to ensure proper credentials.

The dean exploded and said to one of my staff members at the meeting, while pointing right at me, "You guys are running a 'purple polka-dotted' cartel over there in RHS. Did you know that some of your patients are being dropped at our doors as well? How dare you accuse us of this atrocity?"

I was hurt and shocked. I shot back too quickly, "What exactly did you mean by you guys?" A pin dropped, and the meeting ended with the dean excusing himself because of a "headache" with the senator in tow.

A few of their team members remained, and I inquired regarding the patient orphaning. It was true. They were some of our short-length-of-stay patients who didn't qualify. That's right, another investigation. I was a bit late on this one because the local television investigative reporter was already on the doorsteps of our main campus hospital letting the world know, live, that we were responsible for dumping patients and fraud, according to the university, who was strongly considering cutting ties.

Over the next week, I received a lot of lawyer calls from the university and 40-some whistleblower retaliation complaints against me and my team. It was a flood. The doc and many others banded together to fight. Our Region Corporate Officer felt it best to remove me to "reduce the heat", so I got sent home and some of my team too, and here I am.

All the complaints stated "retaliation". I'm no bully. I was just doing my job. The dean seemed like a bully and a bigot. What am I to do now?

Luke

Wow, I thought. Ruth never came up for air, and I was out of breath listening and feeling the escalation in my own body. I tried to comfort her. "Hey, Ruth, friend, you got this."

She interrupted and definitely was crying. "To make things as bad as they could ever be, my dad called yesterday. He has pancreatic cancer, stage 4. I don't know what to do, Luke. I think I'm going to leave RHS. It just makes sense to me. I must be with my dad. I don't have anyone else but him. You know that. I work too hard to meet and keep someone. I don't think there's hope. They always win. They do."

I was stalled but knew I had to say something. So, I blew it. "I am so sorry, Ruth. I could just feel your angst through the phone. Seems we are constantly being reminded these CEO jobs aren't for the weak in spirit. I think your assessment is on point." What possessed me to ask the next question was embarrassing, but I did it. "Have you given any thought to your own biases in this whole thing? I bet you have and you're beating yourself up. Stop that. Good to be introspective, but you're right not to take the blame. I know it is remarkable to have that many complaints, but the investigators should be able to see through that smog. We've got a good law crew here at RHS, too. Glad you're having a bit of a sabbatical. We all could use one every now and then."

Then, just like usual, I made it about myself. "You know, I'm going through something similar. I'm not under investigation... yet. We found through a systems Six Sigma project over $6 million in obligated research funding to a third party that is, well, not easily accounted for. I've brought it to the third party, and they said they were going broke."

I thought to myself, *How could you be bankrupt if you have six million in your accounts from us? Lots of people warning me to pass this one by. I can't. It's probably a matter of time before the fire and brimstone start to fall on me, too. I can't lose all I've achieved in a single swipe like Ruth may. I just can't.*

Just then, my secretary peeked in the door and said, "You have a meeting, and they're waiting."

I told Ruth to hang in there and keep me updated. Then more useless babble came from my lips. "Don't leave. We need you. Our patients need you. You'll get your chance to go back and keep on fighting the good fight. Trust HR. It's a process. We all go through it for the greater good."

What else could I say or do? We hear those words every day, and it keeps us resilient. I need to be resilient. Never enough time in the day. As I gathered my planner and water bottle, I thought how sad she had to buy a burner cell phone to feel safe. Could this happen to me? Or how long before it does? Who or what is next? Should I get a burner phone or even keep talking with her?

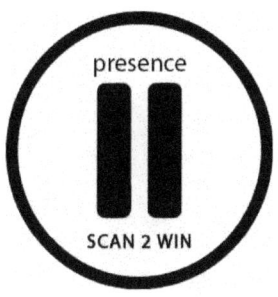

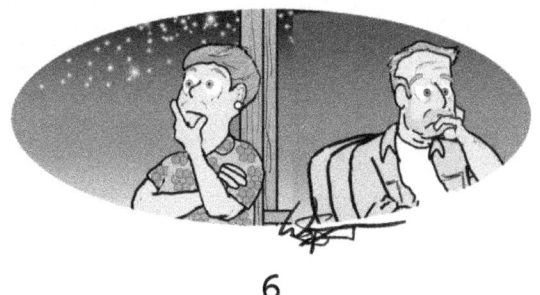

6

Blurred "Code" Grey Lines

Ezekiel and Esther

James 5:16 "Build trust with one another."

Pearl: "Tell the whole story up front, especially when the cat's away."

Ezekiel

Another RHS Leadership week-long course. They are all good, but they seem to blend into one another. I can't stop thinking about how things are going with my team back home. Our last meeting had gone a bit rough with raised voices and subtle, yet mean, talk toward one another and me.

One executive went as far as to blatantly threaten me. "I'm against this and will fight you all the way. Quality management is not that important, nor effective. We do better on our own. Why can't you trust us? We've been doing this for years. You're new. Shouldn't you be watching and learning from us? Just let us be. You'll see."

It's hard to be present here for the training, especially with my cell phone sitting on the table in front of me lighting up with messages from my executive assistant (EA) updating me on the drama back there. Apparently, my chief operating officer (COO) is creating resistance in the finance committee regarding the two critical new positions we need in our quality management team.

I could just drop the hammer and say it shall be because I said so. After all, I am a colonel, for Pete's sake. No, can't do that quite yet. I'm too new to this game and team. I wonder why all this drama. Hmmm.... Things were so much clearer in the military. I miss the Army. What would the general do?

Just then, the instructor caught me daydreaming and called on me. "Hey, why the glum face?" she asked.

I replied, "To be honest, I'm not 100% here. I've got some challenges that seem to be motivated by passive aggressiveness or just plain meanness back at my hospital system. Sorry."

She caringly reminded me we were supposed to be unplugged and to "Trust them to do the right thing while you're here." I felt the prod to turn off my device. It did feel a bit better.

I was sitting next to Esther, who gently nudged me, and she whispered, "Let's do lunch." I agreed.

Most of our courses involving travel are held in cheaper places to save money. The system is cutting staff, as we've got widespread budget woes post-COVID. This one was in the openness of Montana. Who holds a meeting in Montana? Anyway, the sky was truly big. No, enormous.

I tried to send a pic to Miriam, but the majesty was lost in pixel cyberspace. We found a quaint café. Well, not really. It was a tiny mom-and-pop grill. We waited at the door because the small paper sign had red writing which said: "Wait to be seated."

We giggled to ourselves, as there was no one in the place. Well, 15 minutes passed as we watched this one male waiter moving about, fixing tables and not really paying any attention to us. Finally, Esther piped up and beckoned the gent with her smile and kind voice. She joked, "We're here with Jimi Hendrix."

You could tell he had a chip on his shoulder right away as he trotted slowly toward us, muttering one word interrogatively, "Yes?" He was a towering individual and Esther's a smaller framed, older, and humbly dressed lady. I can see her at Woodstock.

I tried to break the ice gently. "We saw the sign and waited. May we be seated? We have limited time for lunch." He rolled his eyes and grunted. He begrudgingly pointed us to a booth near the back and then returned to his nesting-like behavior. Thank goodness there was a QR code to order food, so we did.

A different, very pleasant lady brought our food and addressed Esther respectfully, to see if we needed anything else. We were good, finally having our lunch. Our observation was that customer service was inconsistent, at best. The food was okay.

Esther consoled me. "Hey, I know what it is like worrying about things back home when you're at these meetings. I remember one day very well a few years back. I felt so segregated, and it all was happening while I was at a conference in Florida, time zones away and difficult to be involved. I don't know if you knew, I've got fourteen brothers and sisters. The only crickets I am used to are the ones in the field. And ghosting, what's that? My family is a loud, communicative clan. I don't like quiet when it should not be so.

"There was a patient observed in our hearing clinic. The clerk thought she saw a handgun handle protruding from his jacket pocket. So, she pushed the distress alarm under her desk and a *Weapons Code* was called overhead."

Wow, she sure changed the topic there. A gun?

Esther

The first text I got was, "Active shooter" from my COO. My heart sank and my feet felt numb. This was odd because I had assigned the CFO charge in my absence in written delegation.

I added the CFO and texted back, "Are you all okay?" No response from anyone. I stepped out of the meeting and called my region officer, who knew nothing of the situation. I said, "Let me find out more and I will update you." He agreed.

Finally, about three hours later, I got another text from just the COO. He had purposely removed the CFO. "All good." I was not happy with this *cryptically grey* exchange but felt somewhat relieved. I felt waves of anticipation running over me to hear the after brief. You know, information withholding is a form of bullying and quite disrespectful. I was new, and they were learning to trust me, like your place and team. It led me to think something may have happened to the CFO! Crickets.

Ezekiel

I was perplexed and said, "What on earth?! Were they under duress, limiting them to such mysteriousness? Don't they know we are *ultimately* responsible? Didn't you say it was just a clerk who thought she saw a weapon? Why couldn't, or wouldn't, they tell you?"

Esther

When I returned, it was a Monday, and I requested a meeting for that day or the next. Everyone had conveniently, and conspicuously, conflicting calendars, so it felt to me like they were avoiding meeting with me. I faced my inner bully saboteur and went to go see them. I walked around to their offices, and they all had the same script—it was nothing. "We handled it. You've got a good team here. We didn't need you. The COO is amazing. He said to just ghost you so you could enjoy the conference."

I was new to the facility, like you are now. I tell you, I was at a total loss for words and furious. I had so many emotions and feelings. I couldn't muster a single word, for fear of a war breaking out in me and on them.

This was a unique place. A small city and smaller-minded people yet in a metro. They were not too diverse in their thinking. That's what they accused me of, too. For some reason, they didn't accept my "purple polka-dottiness" and wanted the COO to be CEO. I knew I had to earn their trust, even though they weren't very trustworthy. It was my job.

My EA told me the real story. That she led the 'intervention' while my team stayed out of it. They were critical of her every move and argumentative with her for even being involved. I asked her what "ghosting" is.

"The team is a bit younger than you, ma'am," she said. "It is a thing they do when they don't think it's a good idea to talk to someone because they might get mad." I was at a loss. Crickets, ghosts, oh my. I needed a smoke!

I'll paraphrase what my EA told me: The patient was in the hearing clinic waiting area. He turned out to be a Marine. My EA went with our security to the waiting room to observe. It did appear something was in his lower right pocket. He was wearing a desert tactical vest and sand-colored military boots. He had on a black hoodie over his head and black pants. His appearance on the surface was a bit scary, but also scared and sad. He had his head down, not speaking or looking at anyone. He was tattooed quite a bit, even one on his neck. It was eerie.

My EA felt for him, so she went and sat down beside him. Just sat there. She could see his head turn her way and what appeared to be a tear on his cheek, but they didn't lock eyes yet. She asked him if he was okay and if there was anything she could do to help. She asked him what he was visiting us for and if he served in the military.

He proudly replied that he was a Marine. My EA told him she was in the Coast Guard. He called her a "Coastie", and she called him a "Jarhead." That common ground was helpful.

He was tired of waiting. He had terrible ringing in his ears, couldn't sleep, and had bad PTSD. The poor guy couldn't work or stay in school because he was always late. He had gotten fired that day and his girlfriend walked out on him when he told her. He just needed his hearing aids.

The people here didn't answer the phone. They sent him all over the place. He was here two months ago in the psychology department and stopped by for hearing aids. He still didn't have them. No call, no nothing. He was tired of waiting. So, he was taking matters into his own hands.

It was then she was certain she was seated next to a broken soldier with a gun in his pocket. She asked him if it was okay for a police officer to help them. He agreed.

The officer was amazing. She asked the man if he had seen any signs that prohibited firearms or weapons on our campus. He said he had seen them, and then outright confessed he was carrying a concealed pistol in his pocket but wasn't planning on using it. It was almost like they were friends as he looked up at her and removed his hood respectfully. The officer contained the situation and then called up to the C-suite.

She told me because she was ordered not to bother the CEO, because she's out, to report every move she made to the COO and not her chief or CFO. She whispered to her, "I'm more concerned about reporting this to that bully upstairs than the threat itself." I wondered what's going on in the culture here that an officer is fearful of a showboating leader versus a man with a gun?

Ezekiel

I was enthralled and asked, "What happened next? How did it all turn out?"

Esther

The officer secured the weapon and issued a warning ticket. Then she worked with the hearing clinic, got the hearing aids, hooked him up with the local employment agency, the Veterans Hospital and Psychology. All was good, and she did it all with the help of one talented officer. She then told me the COO chastised her in the hallway because she intervened, too.

BLURRED "CODE" GREY LINES

Well, this patient was well known to my COO, and he, in my absence, bullied over the CFO and told the group, "This guy is crying wolf again. Like all of them. We'd all be better off if they didn't come here for care. They're so much trouble. He's done this before and just wants attention."

The officer later confided in my EA some more. "The last time this patient was called for a response overhead, your COO yelled at me in front of the man in a crowded waiting area. It escalated, and the patient was detained by another officer. I froze in fear because I knew I had no top cover. My captain is friends with the COO and does whatever he is told. I got wrote up for not deescalating the patient and needing an executive to help me do my job."

I may be small, but I wanted to go Incredible Hulk on them. I centered myself and paid attention to what was going on in my stomach, legs, and shoulders. I'm glad I took that presence pause. Later, I did get an opportunity to discuss with the team. But, before that, there was my pompous COO at my door with this pretentious and professional whitewashed humility saying, "Ma'am, do you have a moment? *Your team* would like to talk to you about your lack of trust in them."

Shock is not quite the right vocabulary to use here to describe my cognitive and somatic state of dissonance. My assistant interrupted the exchange where I was about to counsel the COO that the CFO was to be in charge. I wanted to know why he did not follow my orders. Instead, I dismissed the narcissistic COO. He huffed, and I could hear his door slam. Shortly afterward, there was a lot of giggling muffled by his door. My assistant confided that the COO had applied for CEO several times, yet didn't get it due to not being good at honesty and follow-up. The hospital board, as well as corporate, had little confidence in him. Get this, the dude applied for another job and in the background check, they discovered he didn't have a degree. Bye-bye, Mr. McFly.

Ezekiel

Immediately, I felt the empathy between the two of us. Esther has a way about her. It was time to return to the course. My phone was still lighting up. I put it aside. Appropriately, the next lecture was on threat management, of all things.

That evening, back at the hotel, I unloaded the stories of the day on Miriam. She listened intently and wanted to share about her day too. I kept dwelling on it, and she softly said, "I know you're good at what you do, Zeke. You'll figure it out, I'm sure. It's getting late. You need your rest. Remember, you retired once. We're good, so you don't have to do this if you don't want to. I'll support you, whatever." We said our I love you and ended the call.

That was the first time in my career that I felt a bit lonely and dismayed. As I closed my eyes, it dawned on me. I may have just bullied my wife out of her day and into my chaos. I've got to remember to apologize for that. Does this type of drama exist everywhere in RHS? Is anyone immune?

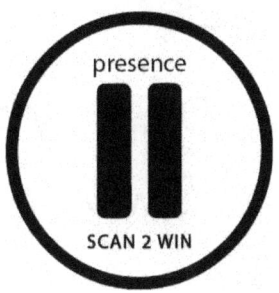

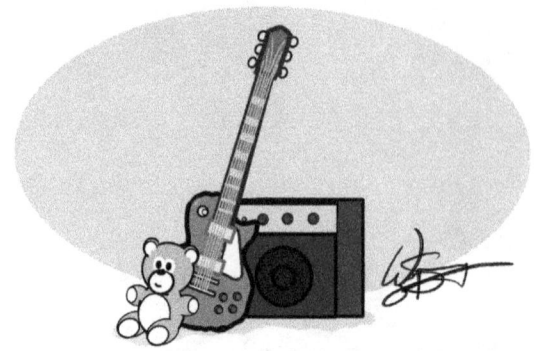

Belle's Diary: Entry Two

Dear Diary, Wow! Married a couple of years! He is so kind. We just had our first little one. It snowed so bad that college classes got canceled. Jazz came home early to find that my water broke!

I'm writing to you from the hospital. There she is in her little incubator at the side of my bed, with that pink sock on her head. She's my princess.

Jazz went home, but now with this storm, it's been three days since he's been able to get back, and they want to discharge me. I'm still upset about last Friday night. Jazz, being a musician, still plays in bands. I don't know how I feel about that. I will tell you I am not impressed with his bandmates' wives.

Jazz is a senior airman, an enlisted man. I never knew what this meant until Friday. I was at the table with other wives, and they were talking about their husbands being "officers" and what their ranks were. Then they got to me. They were complimentary of Jazz's musicianship, but his rank turned them into laughing hyenas. I felt small for myself and for Jazz. They spoke in a snide manner. "Oh, he's enlisted." They slowly left me at the table alone for various excuses. Whatever! I bet their poop still stinks.

I found my joy again, laying peacefully in her little crib. I whispered to her, "Where is your daddy? I want to go home."

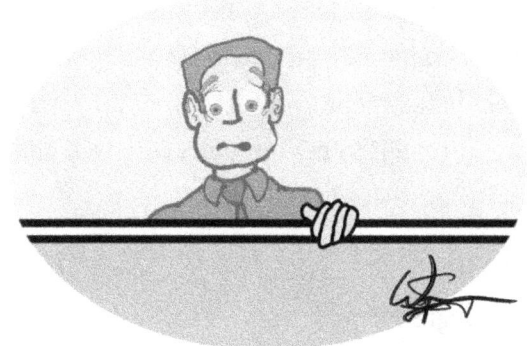

7
Leaving the Scene of a Crime

Ezekiel and Sage

Hebrews 3:13 "Help one another."

Pearl: "See something–say something."

Ezekiel

I texted Sage to see if he had a moment to chat. He quickly responded, as most retirees do. No, I'm not being judgmental, just factual. It was his well-earned freedom, and I was envious, to be honest. Miriam might be on to something. I was relieved he responded. And then my phone rang.

Sage said, "Hey Zeke. How's it going?"

I asked him the same and told him I was seeking some advice on a speech my communications officer had written for an RHS pledge against harassment event later today. I really didn't feel my heart in it. I read it to my secretary as a trial and she didn't feel anything. She advised I rewrite it.

Sage agreed it was a bit cookie cutter and said, "How about I tell you a story of regret?"

I teased him, "Will it be five words... or your advice?" We both chuckled.

Sage

I started my career as a young civilian in the US Navy logistics world before I got into healthcare. I had a cubicle just like everyone else, but mine was just a little bigger, so I had a bit of prestige. Our admin workstation was on the other side of my front cubicle wall, behind the customer service desk. It was tight quarters, but room for a small desk, typewriter, and phone. There were Navy office squids in there too. I was about 25 years old at the time, working on my MBA. They bring in this sharp-dressed sailor, who was an admin for the team. He was cocky, and we were a laid-back shop. At first, I wasn't too sure about this sailor, so I kept my distance. The main supervisor was a civilian grade-12, and the mid-level chief was a 13. I was a 7. The kid out front was an E-3 Navy seaman youngster of low rank.

LEAVING THE SCENE OF A CRIME

Our team worked hard, and we got things to where they needed to be, on time and in the right amount. I had been there several years and was considered part of the family. Weekly, the boss had to report up and our seaman typed the message to HQ because the boss couldn't type. It was a long message, and we had manual IBM typewriters back then. You know what those are? Anyway, it took a long time, like about two hours, to type it with no mistakes and carbon paper. The kid typed well. I always knew it was getting to be the weekend when I would hear his tap, tap, tap and the ring of that carriage return—Ding!

I liked my boss. He was a short, round man and a pear-shaped dude. He had a cool handle-bar moustache he was constantly waxing. More importantly, he laughed like Santa and was really involved in the community through his Free Masons club. He was well liked by our customers, too. Everyone thought he was great, and so did I. His boss pretty much was into his suits and stayed away from all of us out front. I liked it that way, because he wasn't nosing around in my business.

One day, I was in my cubicle and the wall moved in front of me. Then I heard a chair squeaking. I projected over the wall with humor in my voice, "Hey, keep it down to a low roar out there, will ya?"

The kid replied, "Yeah, it's all good." About 30 minutes later, I heard a mumbled voice that sounded like the boss, so I peered out of my cubicle to say hi.

What I saw was disgusting.

Santa was behind the kid, rubbing his shoulders, and there was no light between his roll of belly and the kid's back. The kid was pushed up to his little desk's edge tightly, and the boss was moving himself against him. I quickly darted back to my desk; thankful I wasn't discovered as a peeping tom. Wait, I'm not a peeper, but that was not a good sight. I talked myself out of it; that it wasn't what I thought. I was afraid and my *integrity* failed me. Believe it or not, I'm not proud of this; hence the *story of regret* that I've never told anyone.

What I saw was harassment. Heck, it was an attack. It also went on for almost a year, and then miraculously, the seaman got a promotion and moved on.

I ran into the kid while out on rounds one day and he confessed to me his performance appraisal was lowered by the boss. I sheepishly told him I knew. The kid turned his back and walked away with one finger in the air to me. I deserved it; I suppose. So, Zeke, hopefully my pitfall becomes your pinnacle.

Ezekiel

I thanked the old man and wished him well. I pondered the story of regret Sage shared, and something really kindled inside me. My secretary knocked on the door and said they were ready for me for the pledge. I had no time to edit the speech, so I just went with it from the heart.

Afterwards, my secretary stopped me and said, "Wow, what a speech! The place was riveted. I bet you feel good."

I thought, *I didn't change a thing. I just read from a different lens; maybe because I was still present in Sage's tale of regret.*

Harassment of any kind is not human and should not be. It was a story of abused innocence by power.

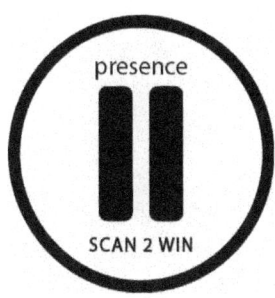

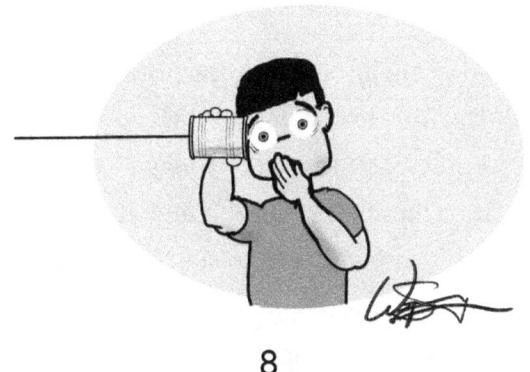

8

Do You Hear What I Hear?

Ezekiel - Self Talk

Romans 12:16 "Be of the same mind to one another."

Pearl: "Be mindful of the telephone game."

What a beautiful night, Christmas Eve. There's something about this season that no other time of year has. Joy, peace, goodwill to all men and family. I'm so thankful for my family. Here we sit, the first time in this church. It's a huge city we now live in, and there must be over 20,000 people in here. Some people are dressed in their Christmas best, some are in jeans, and some are in pajamas. The cool part is everyone is here for the same reason, so it would seem.

The choir is now singing one of my favorite carols. Bing Crosby sang it first, "Do You Hear What I Hear?" As I sing along, I find my mind creeping back to earlier today at the office, and to the past six or so months. I fight the urge to listen to my inner dialogue just a bit, at first trying to stay present here at church of all places; yet it's powerful, and something in the song drove me to these reminiscent thoughts of my failure today.

The scene was my office. The players were my CMO, physical therapy manager (PT), the union president (UN), and our human resources officer (HRO).

The union president requested the meeting because she had received around 30 complaints from within the PT line, of bullying by the line manager and me. I was quite surprised at my involvement. I'm the CEO? Anyway, I listened. I had established a pretty good partnership with the union so far. We were typically on the same page and communicated often and regularly.

I have this wonderful open-door policy, and my secretary does a great job scheduling any staff member for ten minutes with the CEO. Quite often these chats wind up being 30 minutes or so. That's okay with me because I learn so much.

It was about six months ago that the PT manager and I discussed her desire to know more about her staff, to improve the workplace score. She already had a strong patient care line, in my estimation.

She described her concern. "I think my staff might be stagnant, and I know they are hungry for education opportunities. There is a RHS policy now that affords them the ability to advance in specialization and certification. I know we are short on travel funds, but wanted to share with you some of my thoughts about how we could help the stellar rehab staff get even better."

I liked her ideas. She's a sharp one.

In our C-suite private meeting, I pulled her supervisor, the CMO, aside and mentioned the initiative. I also spoke with our chief financial officer (CFO) to see how we might share some discretionary funds with PT to do this great idea. The CMO was super excited and sent an email out to all the rehab front-line staff. I was cc'd on it. I remember telling my CMO to check with their manager first to get the details, because I had only heard ten minutes or so of the idea. I also emphasized that I supported the idea. I told him to iron the details out with his team, then we would review. My CMO is older, and an experienced orthopedic surgeon with over 30 years with RHS—a seasoned professional whom I trusted. I think he just got a bit too excited.

I read that email a few times and felt he had missed the mark. Without taking a single moment to think about it, I marched down the executive suite corridor, with each of my progressive footsteps increasing in veracity and sound level. Miriam tells me I do that sometimes at home.

The CMO popped out of his door smiling, as he always does, and said, "I heard you coming, boss. What's up?"

I laid into him without a single breath taken. "Why would you send this email without talking with me first? I sure hope it doesn't come back to haunt you."

As quickly as I had marched down there, I took a virtual Humvee ride back to my office and slammed my door. As I sat down, I realized what a foolish and mean thing I'd done so spontaneously. I couldn't apologize; I'd gone too far. Still today, especially today, we just pass in the hallway and don't make eye contact. He only sends me cautious emails. We once had been close and easy going.

What happened?

The union president was in rare form today. I really respected her, and we have a strong partnership. But today she was very different, much more animated than usual. Our HRO said she had posted several disparaging things about me on social media. Spitting, I mean, truly spit was frothing from her mouth as she spoke, "It is unprecedented that management would hold a carrot in front of our dedicated bargaining unit and then pull it away like the big bullies you all are. I'm disgusted and quite hurt by this. You need to pay up. RHS must restore all employees to whole."

Well, I've heard that line from her before, minus the saliva. I think she was right this time.

I listened as the employee told their tale. "We love our department. Thank you, Madam Union President, for helping us with this. We were so happy to see the CMO email telling us all we were going to be promoted to the next pay scale level. However, when we started working with our manager and bringing in receipts, we found there were important parts about getting certification, and that we would not be reimbursed for our attendance in the courses, when it was promised to us in the email from the CMO.

"We understand that *you, Mr. CEO Scrooge*, told our manager this was an approved action. We would be promoted, and our cost of education was covered by RHS. So, we did it.

"I spent a lot of money on my new certification, only to discover I will not be reimbursed or promoted. I don't make that much and spent quite a bit of my family's savings, as well as time to do this for the organization and our patients. The least you could do is pay me for my work. We thought you all were our heroes, and then this happened."

It was at that point, I realized why the song had led me into this internal dialogue, and I missed the priest's message, as well as a manger play our neighbor's kids were in. The CMO did not listen to what I told him, and maybe I hadn't listened to what the PT manager was saying, either. Oh boy.

Rewinding now, I hear Charlie Brown's mother mumble, because I'm pretty sure I was formulating what I would say to the PT manager to impress her. Now, suddenly, I'm the bully to these fine and dedicated employees. Worse yet, I realized I can't change a RHS policy. Some of them who were falsely promised will not get the prize and they might be out money. The cat was out of the bag too soon, and now we were trying to corral it.

My verbal vomit justification was, "...a misunderstanding and RHS failed to review the email before it was sent forth."

Well, those words haunt me now.

The union president chewed on it for a second, smiled a Cheshire cat grin, and then blasted me. "Aha! You acted as a mediator/ negotiator between management and my employees. We are the sole representation. You know that! You didn't share that planned email or even talk to us about it. I will be filing a lawsuit."

I could feel my shoulders rising, my teeth clenching, and my gut reeling. She was somewhat right. We didn't act as partners. I jumped the gun a bit and was not very clear, nor did I attempt to be. I thought better of my CMO and PT manager to talk, versus taking my suggestion as a gospel of sorts. My CMO could only cower under HR's glare across the table.

Just then, Miriam nudged me and said, "Earth to Ezekiel! Are you going up for communion? You're holding up our row."

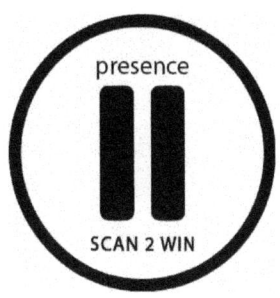

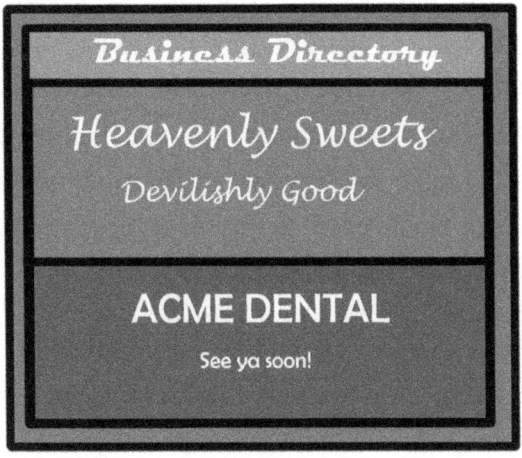

9

Candy and Cavities

Kat and Esther

Romans 14:13 "Do not judge one another."

Pearl: "Just because candy is sweet, doesn't mean you won't get cavities."

Kat

Interviewer: "So Kat, tell us about a time when your emotions got in the way of clear thinking. What was the context? What did you do? How did you feel? What would you do differently?"

I answered incoherently and in a "too much information" format: Not sure if it was the rainy night or the glistening glass of sparkling wine, but something drew me to drag out my middle school yearbook. Ah, the good ole Bobcat days. Go Cats! Go! I was fond of our school mascot, as it matched my name, and I sketched the logo on every one of my spiral notebooks. So, when everyone would cheer, it was like a super affirmation. Not really, but it was cute to me. Kat—Cats!

I was a cheerleader and a good one. We competed at nationals. Didn't win, but hey, we competed and took home a third place. I also was always in the "gifted" groups because of my smarts. So, as I flipped pages through the fifth grade, my eyes and heart stopped dead in their tracks… there she was—that "purple polka-dotted" witch of a girl.

My finger lost grip on the page from the sweat and shaking. She really got to me. I remember it well. Her favorite word was "Why." She would say, "Why is your hair greasy? Why does your mom make you that for lunch? Why do you think you're better than me?" Ugh!

Being in the gifted program and being "pretty" helped me greatly with my teachers, bosses, mentors, etc.… My peers, however, they found ways to blame and discredit me at every opportunity. One instance I remember was in the girls' locker room. She and a couple others shoved me into my locker and closed the door. I'm a woman now, but I think back to that story of Joseph and how his own brothers threw him in a pit and sold him off to the Egyptians. Dad was loaded. I mean, he had wealth. Both he and my mom were up there in politics. My youth was a lot like that and even until today, I've been an outsider. What happened today was just plain crushing and gross.

BUZZZZ! What was that? Oh, it was my alarm. That was a dream? Not my favorite dream. Thank God that was not a real interview! I didn't make any sense. Why can't I shake the nightmare when he took my life away?

I needed to get ready. Big day ahead—the Young Professional Women's Summit panel with a woman healthcare CEO, Esther, from the esteemed RHS. Her biography is amazing. I couldn't wait to hear her presentation and ask a few questions.

DING! I pulled my steaming cup of coffee from the microwave, went to the fridge and poured half of the sweet Italian creamer into my first morning java. Oh, and I couldn't forget that extra shot of pumpkin spice syrup! So nice! Then, off I went.

The registration table was typical, with the "My Name is:" sticker that only stays on through the first ten minutes of the morning and the rest of the day you're trying to figure out how to keep it on; or is it on the right or left? So many choices.

I had an assigned seat. I sat at my table and there were some wonderful women there. We made small talk about the prestigious Esther we'd all heard so much about. Her official photo was faded and pretty jacked up, if you ask me. Someone could have done better with it. Anyway, there was an empty seat at our table and some strange lady plopped down. I was like, *seriously?!*

She was short and meek in stature—maybe 4 foot and 90 pounds. Her hair looked like she didn't own, or even know, what a brush is. Her top was so oversized and drab it just fell like old, moldy fall leaves from a grand-sized oak tree, and her glasses were refurbished soda bottle ends. She had a nose like a beak, and right next to it was a sizeable mole. She looked oddly like John Lennon. (I'm being descriptive, not derogatory.) The rest of us were well kept. Of course, I was the prettiest. I must be.

The woman said a quick, "Good morning, ladies." She must have struggled with this silly sticker name tag too, because she wasn't wearing one. I offered to get her a name tag. I had an ulterior motive—coffee and sugar. She thanked me, so off I went.

I took as many as sugar packets as possible. I popped like ten into my pocket, balanced the two coffee cups, and sauntered to the table. I also came back with a marker and pen, and she said, "My handwriting is not so good, due to my eyesight and these thick glasses. Would you be a dear and write Esther on the tag?"

Would I?! So, I introduced myself as Kat, a federal court lawyer. She said, "You're very kind, Kat, and pretty. I like your outfit. I can never pick anything out for myself."

The Master of Ceremonies called the honor guard forward and the National Anthem began playing. She told us where the "housekeeping" things were, like the ladies' room, and that they had dedicated two men's rooms for overflow. There were no men in the building, nor in the summit, but there was no way I was entering the urinal capitol. I was secretly safe with no men there. As the words of our country's anthem washed over me, the part about "the perilous fight" rang true to me after yesterday. *Ick, put that out of your mind, Kat, and be present at this summit. Does "perilous" have to be repeated over and over?*

The MC read her biography, and it was long. Esther sat next to me until the MC was 100% completely done. She waited until all the applause had ended before she stood. Like a squirrel on the forest floor, I noticed her right eye was on me like that of a barn hawk, as I added another sugar packet to my already cooling coffee. She was not very ambulatory, had a cane on her left side, and slowly waddled to the podium while we all were silent, waiting for her to begin.

Esther started, "Good morning. Or is it? Yes, it is. Every morning is good when you make it that way. Ladies, I've never been the pretty one. I've never been asked to a prom. I've never married. Never walked along a sunset beach romantically with a partner. I've never missed any of that, either." Then she sang a line from a Miley Cyrus song about buying flowers for herself.

The crowd erupted with laughter and cheers as she had just eloquently and effectively broken the initial "judge a book by its cover" adage we all were fighting off in our heads and hearts.

Esther continued, "I always had a strong interest in computers and business. Guess that's why I have 3 MBAs, 2 PhDs, and am a medical doctor of psychiatry, which you've all read in my bio. And if not, you can." The crowd applauded. She waited again and looked downward at her shoes.

When she looked up, the glare from her glasses shot little colored prisms all around the room. It was surreal and adorable.

Esther

Life and work for the not-so-pretty girl is a monumental peak. Some just give up trying to climb and take a back seat job. I didn't do that. I may have at first, but it really brought me out of my shell when a boss of mine, a woman, tore into me one day about my appearance and my "executive presence".

Now, I must tell you that I did not live a lavish youth. My dad was a middle school custodian/bus driver and Mom stayed home with us 14 kids. We didn't have money, and we had clothes from Goodwill, but they were just fine. I never got teased in school, either. My mom was handy, and she made some of the clothes we wore. It was good back then and simple. As an adult, young professional woman, however, it has been a brutal journey.

I said to the ladies, "I digress. I'm here today to stimulate you, encourage you, uplift you, give you a big ole fashioned Rah, Rah, Sis, Boom, Bah speech, right?" I lowered my voice, took off my glasses, and said, "Do you want that, or do you want the truth? Your choice. Can we get real?"

The crowd leaned in toward me, and softly whispered in low tones, "Yes."

My mom would tell us stories, and we know the power of stories, so allow me to tell you mine. It was my first CEO job, not with RHS. I had worked my way up and there I was. This was nearly

25 years ago, ladies. So, it is possible that the culture was a bit different then. But is it?

I had worked my first 90 days, and it was time to meet with my boss. She was a Barbie look-alike mixed with a Hillary Clinton type. She was older than me and wore braces, and she likely had stock in plastic and Botox! My boss was a barracuda. No, you don't cross a woman like her. I saw her crush a male CFO in a closed-door meeting and thought, *I sure hope I'm never on that side of her.*

So, she began our meeting going over my hospital's improvement in metrics since my arrival, and all was stellar. She even said that she did not expect movement, as this hospital was a good ole boy network of people who had been there for years. She asked me what my secret was.

I blushed and glowed at the same time and replied, "I strove to drive quality and a safe place to speak up and involved all key stakeholders in decision-making, made friends with the union, and attended service events. Blah, blah, blah…"

The crowd laughed, but I broke the laughter when I told them, "She stopped me and said this, 'Well, it sure ain't your looks, honey.'"

Kat

Silence. I was like, *where's the oxygen?* The crowd deadened with an eerie stillness. I am certain I heard someone's stomach rumble and groan. Some were tearful. Some apologized out loud. Chairs squeaked as we all shifted our physical postures, trying to find that comfort that just wasn't there. It felt like all women were just attacked. I felt my history, and yesterday, all over again, too.

Esther said something next I'll not forget soon. "I told her just because candy is sweet doesn't mean you won't get cavities!"

There was an immediate standing ovation. She cautioned us not to revel in her resorting to bullying, as she called it. We all slumped back into our chairs with the gentle nudge of her remarkable integrity revealed and grace.

Esther

Of course, I was shocked, hurt, dismayed, dismantled and mad. She didn't know me! How could she? She was so tied up in her Barbie collection. Then my boss started using words like "executive presence failure". She went on to describe it: "One must dress for success. Don't let anyone get too close. Be vocal. Don't be timid. Get what you want and know what you want, so they know you're going to get what you want because you want it. For goodness' sake Esther, I'm paying you good money. Get some nice clothes and go to a salon. Your work is average to good, but your executive presence is absent, and you will fail soon enough because of it."

I know, right? What a load of malarky!

I went home that night, destroyed. I drove by a few boutiques and popped into one. There were no other ladies in the boutique but me and a pretty little thing shuffling about, tucking in sleeves and straightening mannequins. She caught view of me and said, "Um we don't offer discounts in our posh shop." I tore out of there, got in my car, and lit a smoke.

Kat

From her appearance, I wondered a moment if that was tobacco.

Esther

I tried and failed, just like my boss said I would. That was a long drag on that smoke; but I gathered my wits, called my mom and she said, "Go back in there and be nice to the youngling. Then tell her where your bank account is at and put her on the spot. Then you ask her to help you find a nice dress and shoes. Be nice about it."

The crowd, beside itself, collectively asked me, "Did you?"

I answered, "Yes, I did."

I never wore that dress to work, but I did wear it home on Thanksgiving and Mom loved it. What I'm saying is, I learned to be "present" and "be" with who I am, and what I feel, and how I show up. When people say things like this to me now, I recall my independence in buying a dress I liked, but controlling my response to the point that I didn't need to wear it to work. About two years into that assignment and getting only fully successful ratings from my Barbie boss, she was investigated for having been involved with human sex trafficking. Another charge against her was her involvement with a promotion of a male employee who she was a bit too friendly with. She was fired.

I was sad for her, but there's karma for ya, ladies.

Before I close, I would like to recognize Kat. She's a fine lady who also happens to be a federal lawyer. Kat, thank you for getting my name tag for me.

In closing, I wrote Barbie a note. Are you curious?

Kat

Of course we were!

Esther ended her speech with, "Just because the candy is sweet, doesn't mean you won't get cavities."

What a speech! We all applauded, and then it was time for the panel. Nope, they switched it to small groups, not a full-on panel. More intimate that way.

Back at our table, Esther looked at me, and as if she had crawled into my mind space, said, "Tell us all about it." I was surprised, but she saw right through me. I could no longer hide the paradox in my head and heart and added the last of my sugar packets to my already empty coffee cup. That nightmare. Why me? Why him?

I told them all how the day before I had been at work with a male junior law partner. He's just gorgeous. I mean, I could build picket fences with this smart and good-looking man.

He said, "Hey Kat, it's just us two here in the office today. How about we get some lunch?" I thought about it. He's two people away from my chain of leaders, he's not my supervisor, we hardly work together... Yes, I accepted his kind invitation with a few butterflies in my tummy. I don't give in easily. I've got a history with men who took advantage of me. So I'm careful. We went in separate cars, so I met him at this deli about a mile away from our courthouse.

The waiter hadn't even brought us water when he looked across the table at me, smiled and said, "So, Kat, does size really matter?"

I dug for something to say and, well, here's what I came up with: "I don't poop where I eat."

I felt like I was in fifth grade and kind of wanted to crawl back into my locker. Maybe this is what that nightmare was all about this morning? Esther reached over and patted me on the hand and said, "There's more?"

I acknowledged there was. I told the group how when I was in the gifted class, there was a girl who kept going to the teacher asking why I got an A, even if she got one too. She also would jump in line for project partner selections and made a point of getting with my best friend. I was often left alone to do the project, or with the teacher. She would laugh and point at me, too. In fact, my mom found out from the teacher that the girl's mom would also call my teacher, wanting to know about my progress.

The teacher probably felt sorry for me and wanted to get to the bottom of it. What she did follows me to this day. She called my mom, her mom, my best friend's mom, and all the girls together for a lunch. At that lunch, she said, "We all know that Kat is sensitive, and I would like you all to start playing well together. No more stealing partners. No more asking me about grades for someone that is not your own child." It was embarrassing and the bullying increased. The lies and teasing continued when no one was looking.

So, at work, I don't let people get close to me. I dress conservatively to not draw attention. I keep to my faith and my business. I have always striven to support my bosses and teachers and do well at it. In fact, I've received promotions because of my quality work. Legitimately promoted. I earned them.

What happened after that "lunch" was not good either. No one at the courthouse, especially the women, would talk to me. I often found myself in the breakroom all alone. Yesterday, one of the senior law clerks to the judge came to my desk and asked me. "Why did you get this job, anyway? He's such a nice man. He was just trying to help you. How could you?"

I thought, *I'm about to be fired*, as I noticed the crystalizing sugar in the bottomless coffee cup.

CANDY AND CAVITIES

Esther leaned back and said, "This is why I didn't bully my boss back. Karma, baby, it comes around. But when karma is not closing on our timeline for justice, we sure do get down on ourselves, don't we? My boss was right about one thing, ladies: executive presence. And she didn't have any. It's not what she said, however. It is how I have been honed through my life experiences, and how well I know my body's somatic responses when presented with an opportunity to respond freeze, fight, or flight."

The hawk in Esther opened its beak, like it was about to devour me. She counseled, "Ladies, sweetness from sugar is a crutch, and can be a killer. I spell sugar S U G A R."

We all scowled, especially me.

Esther said, "Your Senses can Unhinge you, your presence and health. It goes to your Gut and wreaks havoc on your digestive system and your lady-like figure. Worst of all, it affects your Awareness, brain function, cognition, and can be quite addictive. Guess what else?" She paused for a moment, then added, "It may lead to Real problems, like insomnia, inflammation, diabetes, and wow, does it power stress."

I piped up. "Like smoking, Ms. Esther?"

She was quick on the draw, and said, "I didn't qualify if that smoke was from tobacco, now, did I?"

Esther's talk about sugar caused me to hold back the rest of what I was going to say. What I hadn't told them is how my dad's judge friend assaulted me by the pool house after dad got me that summer job at the court. Why did I ever become a lawyer? I thought to myself, *the "Perilous Fight."* Keep going, girl.

I thanked Esther for making me feel liked. She winked at me.

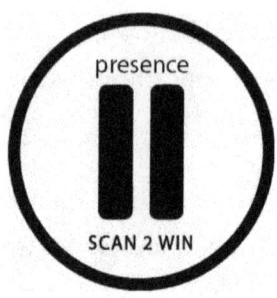

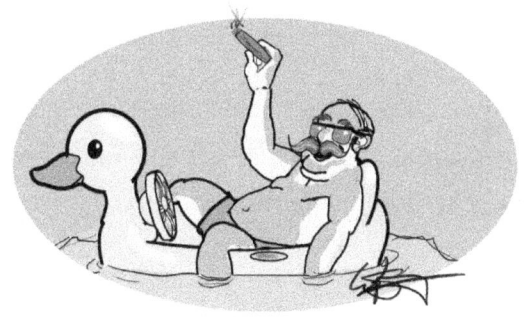

10

Too Sexy for My Shirt

Ezekiel, Miriam and The Honorables

Philippians 2:3 "Be not conceited toward one another."

Pearl: "The least important word is 'I'"

Ezekiel

It was a twist, but we opted out of our normal vacation to the islands. Instead, our nephew John, a law clerk, invited us to a new vacation spot in the South where he and his family moved. They always joined us on the trips, and we enjoyed their company so much. This time he had just started and was about a year into his new job. He shared with me that his judge and team were not the fondest of him and were bullying him quite a bit. It had all started with the "Keurig." He said he needed us to come there, as he might get called to work.

(Don't tell anyone, but John is our favorite nephew—uh, wait, we only have one, and yeah, he's a lawyer and an OEF/OIF Marine veteran!) We're so proud of him. So, we mixed it up and went to John's new home. I can only imagine how a coffee machine and bullying are correlated.

We got a rental car from the airport and headed into town. It was a quaint, southwestern long main drag adorned with juicy, blooming flowers of all colors. There were red, white and blue ribbons and flags with local veterans' pictures on every light pole. An impressive little American town.

John told us where his courthouse was. It was the next left turn. The sound of the turn signal clicking was perfectly in time with our normal heart rates until we saw it. Abel, our hockey player, remarked, "It's a sieve!" Sieve is a word that means to sink the puck into the net when a goalie misses a shot and someone on the other team scores. It's a slang form of accepted sports bullying of goalies. Everyone except the goalie likes to chant it. I couldn't agree more with his assessment. It was something to behold.

There was no other word than sieve.

It was a paradoxical irony before us. The sign made of granite and gold lettering read "Justice Here." The courthouse was set back on the circular drive. There were churches next to it, but both were falling apart, and the pavement was so cracked and dry. Tumble weeds bounced about, as if chasing each other, because there was nothing else to do for entertainment. The Methodist church had become a monument to vines.

Then there was the centerpiece—the town courthouse. Grey (or maybe they were red) bricks, but they were very old. It appeared the windows had wilted from the heat, and they were misshapen, yet clinging in their frames, like loose teeth about to fall out with the slightest bit of encouragement. There were two shiny marble pillars on the steps, which seemed to be freshly polished.

We decided to go pick up John's kids and go directly to the park to go for a dip. Abel stayed back and went to a bar to get a cold one. He's really headed down a bad path since the whole sports thing didn't pan out. Miriam always seems so distant when this happens. Sometimes she even lashes out at me for something not related, like my growing belly. She's got to be thinking something deep. She never talks about it. He drinks a lot—we pray a lot. You can't be too much of a parent when they're in their late 20s. Just pray. Abel's a good human and good things will come soon enough. I sure hope he moves out of my basement. Whoops, that slipped out. I'd miss him so much.

Finally, vacation! It was a balmy 110 degrees in the shade. The palm trees wept in sync with the bad Caribbean music playing through those little horn speakers, and the pool reflected the mid-day sun's brilliance. Miriam smirked. "Honey, not quite the islands. Ha."

Miriam and I got in line with the kids to go into the water park. What a life. I'm so blessed with my family all around. We got our things—everyone did. While we waited to get our tickets, it was impossible not to notice the man in front of us holding what appeared to be a large yellow duck with built-in seats and cup holders. This thing had a mounted fan. It was like the king of floaties, if you ask me. I may have had a slight case of floatie envy.

Now, describing this man will pale compared to the actual life event, but I'll give it a whirl. He was short in stature. The man was as round as he was tall. He sported a mean comb-over of about three lines of greased black hair. His complexion was pitted and worn. His eyelids were multiple. He had a boisterous and authoritative voice. His countenance was serious and almost regal. He appeared to have a manicure on both his toes and hands.

His towel had embroidered initials on it: "FHZIII". The towel was white, but he was paler than the towel. He turned around and said, "You folks go ahead now. See, I'm a local. You go enjoy my park. You might see my name on the big sign as you enter. I'm the major contributor." As he wiggled his unlit fat cigar, he winked. "Glad to see tourists. I need new blood in my town."

I asked him, "Sir, where can I get one of those floaties?"

He bellowed, "My boy, this is a custom-made aqua cruiser; not just a floatie."

I said, "Oh," as my eyes slightly widened. We moved ahead and Miriam thanked him as she turned to me with that telltale eye roll and look. I knew she was not impressed. I am quite familiar with that look.

We got settled in, and John texted me saying he had a conundrum, and he and his wife would join us as soon as he was clear. I texted back, "No worries. We are at the park, and it is very hot. Please bring sunscreen."

Ahhhh... finally, we sat in our little cabana next to the pool, watching the kids splashing and sliding. Just as we finished putting on our sunscreen, the same man with his wife took a commanding roost in the next cabana. He again bellowed, "Hey friends. Glad to see you got the good seats here. This is the top spot in the park. It is our spot. If I'm not making wrongs right, we're right here." He turned toward his wife and said, "Now dear, put some more of that deep tan lotion on me, and don't try to trick me with that screen stuff. I know you like your marshmallow lightly browned."

I was sure Miriam vomited in her mouth. I got a bit choked up, too. What an image!

"Oh, balderdash. Why can't these kid lawyers get anything right?"

His wife patted him, continuing the arduous chore of spreading oil into his ape-like hairy back. She said, "You're relaxing now. Leave it."

He obliged with a "Yes, dear." It sounded like she was commanding a little bull doggie. Leave it?

A few moments passed, and we realized this man was bent on having a conversation with us that he would broker. So, the journey began. He asked what I do for a living and Miriam kicked me under the wicker table, so I said, "I'm an administrator. How about you?"

That was all it took. He opened wide and started a bluster like a tornado tale all about himself. Remember that Toby Keith song?

Well, there's another song by the Turtles called "Happy Forever" that some lawyers had changed to "Appointed Forever" in satire. John sent us a link a while back. It was funny.

Unbelievably, this guy answers me with: "I am THE HONORABLE FRANCIS H. ZINGLEMEISTER, THE THIRD, THE FEDERAL DISTRICT JUDGE. That's who I am and what I do. I make wrongs right. JUSTICE HERE, I say. I am the two pillars on the courthouse here. I love my town, and I keep it. It is my job to do it, and I do it. My friends call me (insert dramatic pause here) 'The Honorable.'"

His wife acknowledged him, saying, "The Honorable and I have been together for 51 years of blissful marriage. I'm so proud of him. He has a hallway filled with pictures of all the young lawyers he has taught. They buy their own frames and pictures and beg him to add them to his wall of mentees. He's such an example to so many."

Then my lovely wife looked at him and said, "I see the monogram on your towel matches your husband's. How cute." I kicked Miriam under the table that time.

He interrupted again and sang a verse from the satire version of the song John sent us. It was déjà vu in a terribly creepy way. He seemed to believe it all. The gist of the song was that everyone should imagine him as a god, just because he was a federal district judge. He ended with a line about being "appointed forever".

This time, I beat Miriam to the punch. "Wow! Forever is a long time. Congratulations." He glowed.

Then he and his wife set sail in the yellow duck, but not too quickly. My wife said in the kindest way, "Nice meeting you, Francis and wife!" Nope. I didn't kick her. We toasted our lemonades.

A few hours had gone by in and out of the pool, making sure we had sufficient sunscreen, as it was a blazing sun. John could not join us, but wanted to talk on the phone. I called him.

John told me that because he was on vacation, he didn't get something done and had to work on it. He said his boss had texted him not the nicest of messages, but he was a "big boy and would deal with it." He asked how the kids were doing. I told him we were having a ball, and we'd be back at his place in about an hour, and we hung up. I wondered if Francis... nah.

The duck beached upon the edge of the pool and "The Honorable" approached. He was frantically sketching something on a pad of paper. I tried not to look, but it was like a cartoon of some sort, yet looked oddly familiar. My wife noted that too.

He and his wife were giggling in a somewhat sinister way. Just then, my phone lit up with a pic from my nephew. It was a cartoon drawing of John. He said his boss was going to publish it in a magazine and put it as his picture in the hall of mentees at the courthouse.

I was too late. Miriam had already gone in for the kill. She said, "Francis, that is an amazing talent you have there. It almost looks like our nephew. John is a lawyer, too, and lives here in town. Maybe you know him?"

I've never seen two people move so fast. They deserted the park and left the duck without another word.

We got back to John's home, and he and I had a moment to review the day.

John

On my first day on the job, the judge and his staff encouraged me to ask questions about anything and assured me they were there to help me. The next morning, I asked for help with a coffee machine and that triggered a lot of teasing and exclusion from the people. Substantiative legal questions were even more negatively received. I couldn't even do my job because all the needed support was pulled like a carpet from under me. Felt like one strike and I was out. But not just out of the batter's box—out of the realm of even minimal decency.

The judge is particular and has this hallway filled with framed pictures of every law clerk he'd ever had. It's his personal trophy wall. My integrity kept me apart from that wall, so I delayed it a bit. Now this? Who draws a cartoon and threatens to publish it because you didn't get a photograph at your own cost and put it up? I have messed up. I came in less prepared than other clerks and had to ask questions that they did not. They also appeared not to make too many mistakes, if any at all. The belittling and sarcasm didn't elevate me. I just don't get why the mockery? What did I do or say outside of seeking help?

The judge took everyone to lunch, and I said jokingly, "Like you're going to get positive feedback on this lunch on your appraisal from me!" That probably could have been done better, or not at all. I really think I'm about to be fired. And without his recommendation, what will I do?

Ezekiel

I knew in my heart the reason we drove by that courthouse was to share these final words with John, and I was inspired to do something about this bullying thing. I planned on talking with Sage about it on our next call.

"John, if you close your eyes and be present with how your courthouse looks compared to how the town is, what do you see?"

He replied, "Dead, drying out, no sign of hope, and it is the same on the inside. Every day I go into work with a better attitude, and it seems like I'm just there for the sentencing."

There's a saying, "Some can knock you down a staircase and you feel lifted up. Others just knock you down."

"Uncle, there's a bit more. The judge won't talk about this openly (hard to believe), but he has a daughter who is 'purple polka-dotted' with a disability. Sometimes, I overhear him venting to the 'cool staff' about how heartlessly people write her off without helping. He is lacking self-awareness that he is bullying lots of people himself. I kind of feel for him in a weird way."

We all retired for the night. Miriam leaned over and said, "Great day at the park. What a blowhard of a bully. But you know what?"

I replied, "What?"

"He's going to look like a lobster with extra blisters in the morning."

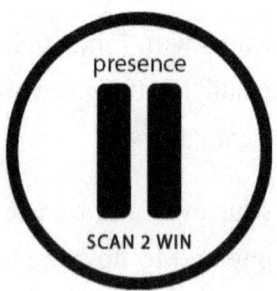

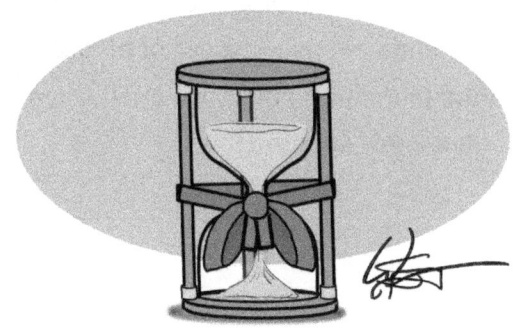

Belle's Diary Entry 3

Christmas Gift of Time

Dear Diary, I really concentrated on what to get Jazz for Christmas this year. I thought, well, it's been almost 25 years now since we've been married. Kids are grown and doing well. His career has soared, and we've moved two times now in the past three years. In retrospect, it's been okay. Sometimes I feel Jazz is so different. At work, he's the epitome of an energetic, thoughtful, and engaged man. At home, I can't lie; dinner tonight was a bit frightful. Every time I looked up to see him, he was either playing with his dinner or staring into it. I spoke, but I'm sure he wasn't hearing. I sense time is getting away from us. We are contemplating the biggest move of our lives maybe, and his career. When he talks about it, he's excited and I feel the same. When he has downtime, he is almost catatonic. He sleeps a lot and seems like he always has a headache. Hmmm, what do I get him? An ad popped up on my Bible app, and it was an hourglass. Unassuming, about seven inches in height, with its glass tube pinched in the center and sparkling white sand. It had a nice wood and brass construction, too. It hit me—I'll give him time. My time, his time, and time for life to pause and be present in the good things. I miss the sweet tones of his acoustic guitar. It just hangs in the humidor he built. He cried when we opened his gift. I sure hope this does the trick.

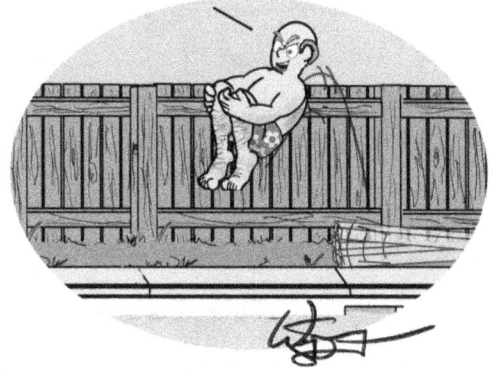

11

Desperate Times - Drastic Measures

Ezekiel, Nabal, and a Line Manager

1 Thessalonians 5:13 "Live in peace with one another."

Pearl: "You're always on stage."

Ezekiel

I thought to myself, *Whew! Saturday, what a week. I'm so glad to be here on the sun porch, looking out at the sparkling pool and watching an old re-run of Columbo before the social chaos starts. I love how that guy rubs the back of his head in subtle humility and then drops the mic on criminals. "Uh, ma'am, just one more thing... when did your husband buy those knives?" What style. Wish I could do that at some board meetings. It will be good to have some friends over today for the pool party. Although we live in the Southwest now, we still have lots of friends who are Southeast baseball fans, and today we're celebrating the big win. What's this?*

Miriam called to me, "Hey, babe! Come in here quick. Something terrible has happened again. There's a breaking news report from the resort area we're headed to next week. I think it's about our team winning the World Series somehow."

The news anchor announced, "We interrupt your normal programming, as we are tracking yet another mass shooting in the southeastern part of the state. It appears that during the parade and festivities celebrating the recent World Series Championship, that four perched sniper gunmen and one woman in the crowd, armed with a handgun, opened fire into the crowd approximately 30 minutes ago, wounding an unspecified number of people. It is alleged the woman shooter was wearing the opposing team's hat. It is unclear as police and other first responders gather wounded what the ultimate outcome will be. The area is now secured by SWAT and FBI.

"A spokesman for Major League Baseball stated, 'There is a shock the size of ten Category 5 hurricanes in our communities today. Senseless acts and senseless losses. We need gun control or something. America's pastime has been violated in a way never seen before. Our hearts are with all involved and their families, as we wait for authorities to right this wrong. We do know we've lost the MVP, and several other players are receiving medical care for serious gunshot injuries they received during the parade. Countless fans, children, and adults have been injured as well.'"

The anchor continued. "Among those wounded and killed, we are now hearing the local veterans' hospital and State Home for Veterans had a group of nearly 200 at the parade. This just coming in... there are several decorated veterans who have been killed or injured. We'll keep you updated as developments come in. If you are traveling, or in the area, please consult with local authorities on what areas are currently closed. Do not go downtown except for official business. Homeland Security Authorities currently do not suspect terrorist activity."

Just then, our doorbell rang, and our friends started coming into our home. Some knew about the shooting, while others were just finding out. Kind of put a damper on our party mood. We consoled one another, and we all slowly relocated out to the pool, and I checked on the smoker and grill. It only took one cannon baller to get the party started on a very sad day.

I snuck away to call my new buddy, Nabal, to see how things impacted being they are in that city. "Hey man, how ya doing?"

Nabal said, "Thanks for calling. Obviously, I don't have a lot of time. We set up Incident Command and are assisting as best as we can. I'm at the hospital with my EA and emergency manager. The rest of the C-suite is vacant and not reachable yet—some team! Maybe they were there. I don't know because none of them are answering. The assistant CMO is on site, however, driving nurses and docs in the ED, readying for the trauma. Our local partner hospitals and the VA are swamped, so we are pretty much on our own here as casualties and wounded pour in for care.

"Man, they shot kids. It's a state of disbelief, man. This is horrible. Ironically, last month we held a successful active shooter tabletop scenario with the whole community. RHS really shined."

I agreed and offered if he needed staff, we would do what we could on our end to assist despite the budget. I told him call at any time and thanked him. He's had a rough time of it over the past year with team issues, inspections, lawsuits and the like. Now this.

Back out to our friends. The pool was frothy with bubbles from all the activity, and towels spread about on loungers and the decking. Kids were screaming, laughing, and lots of chatter. As I appeared, they all stopped and wanted an update. I shared what Nabal had told me of their horror, and our pastor offered to pray. It was somber, yet impressive, how nearly 40 people and kids just stopped for silence and prayed. I thought to myself, *there's a lot of different people and faiths who all are fans of the team, yet here today this unites us deeply.*

Miriam smiled and scurried about, tending to the snacks while talking with others, spreading what joy she could. She's such a good hostess. We brought out the pulled pork and everyone feasted.

DESPERATE TIMES – DRASTIC MEASURES

As the sun set, the crowd thinned a bit, but still 20 or so remained. It was a great get-together. I know I'm not supposed to fraternize, but life is life, work is work, and everyone needed this let-your-hair-down moment. This was somewhat of a distraction—certainly bittersweet. Honestly, how important are sports, considering this tragedy that keeps happening in so many parts of our lives and country?

As the evening deepened, Miriam and I sat along the edge of the pool, relaxing and conversing with another couple about their recent travels to the Caribbean. On the opposite side of the pool was one of our guests, a super guy who joined RHS about a year ago. He just started out loud with a story about work. He and another guest were commiserating culture. It was easy to overhear. It sounded like a recent personnel matter—no names. I tried to block it out as background venting. This man is a war hero. He was a retired officer/pilot in the Air Force who flew top secret missions that resulted in terrorist leader captures/kills. He'd give you the shirt off his back, so humble and kind. Still... it got a bit in the way of my "plausible deniability", as I could wind up being responsible for discipline or testimony in court.

Anyway, the conversation went something like this:

Line Manager

We must stop these people from thinking they can just go shoot others. We've been struggling with an employee whose performance is not good. He's got skills, but just not the right ones for his position and he knows it. He's a bit on the odd side.

His teammates aren't terribly fond of him. In fact, they're scared of him. He struck one of them physically and tore apart some furniture last month. He's an intimidating figure of a soldier who always wears his ball cap reversed, with a tuft of his long, red hair sticking out of the hat. No one really knows what's going on. He is a veteran, but he also is not showing up for work a lot lately. Anyway, HR tells me we're close now in the documentation process and should let him go. My assistant manager is not ready to do that and wants to meet once more with HR and include me. That was two weeks ago. We met.

So, we sit down and review his case file, and it is time for my assistant manager and me to have that important talk with the guy. Being the manager, I don't directly supervise him. My assistant does, and he's been keeping me up on how this fellow is failing and causing a psychologically unsafe workplace. My assistant manager is a seasoned leader, and he's tough to rattle.

He told me he's worried for this employee, because he's an Army sniper and was in combat. People are afraid of him. What he might do. He talks about having the "tools and skills" to mess people up, as he puts it. Intruding, HR pipes up and dumps on us that the guy's wife has been calling them, wanting to know why his supervisor allows the bullying by his peers. She is demanding they do something about it, or she will expose it to media. It was then we knew that he hadn't told his wife about his ongoing performance issues or conduct and that he was about to lose his job. He was counseled recently that he was on his last strike and probably should start looking for other opportunities.

Well, last week he and his wife started posting on their social media pages that they're going to "...*expose and get even with the bullies taking our life from us at RHS. If we can't have a family, neither will they.*"

So they basically threatened my assistant's family. That's not something you do with my assistant! He's super family oriented. My assistant called me that evening at home, quite upset. He said he didn't feel safe and had called the police to get a restraining order. I tried my best to bring him in off the ledge. I thought that went okay.

Ezekiel

I looked at Miriam. She just shook her head and said, "Stay here, Zeke." We were intently eavesdropping. At that point, it was unavoidable. You know how hard it is to be listening to one conversation but really interested in another?

Line Manager

The next morning, the employee showed up outside my office with his voice raised at my secretary, saying, "I know you're all watching me and have my home bugged. Don't you know I lost my son and my dad in the last year?! Do you even give a hoot? Everyone is prejudiced against me because I'm 'purple polka-dotted'. Well, the time is now, and I am about to show RHS a thing or two. Shock and awe, baby. You go tell that manager of yours!"

I was on the phone, so I couldn't get out there fast enough to relieve my secretary from the onslaught. When I did get to her, she was broken down crying, and asked to go home because she was scared.

This whole thing with people showing up and shooting others has got to stop. We've got to take matters into our own hands. I'm an American too. I wasn't proud, but I was scared for my family. My assistant and I both decided we would concealed carry our own pistols to work the day of the removal. It seemed like a good idea at the time. I didn't know what that guy or his wife were capable of, and I went into my innate officer mode from the sand trap to protect those who I led and my family. I realize now that we took weapons on hospital property and probably would have lost our jobs or still could. Maybe that wasn't smart.

Ezekiel

Okay, now that I've heard this, or did I? Really, you brought a gun to my hospital?! What would I have done? Not that.

He then said, "But these desperate times call for drastic measures."

It was too late to stop him as he picked up steam. "Just look at what happened at the parade today. My son might be at that parade down there, and we haven't heard from him yet. I guess that's why I did it."

Miriam and I looked at each other—we didn't say anything. No, not a word. Shock and awe.

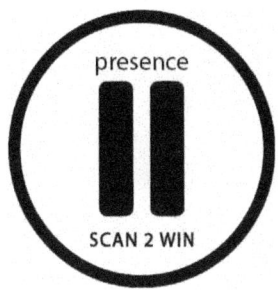

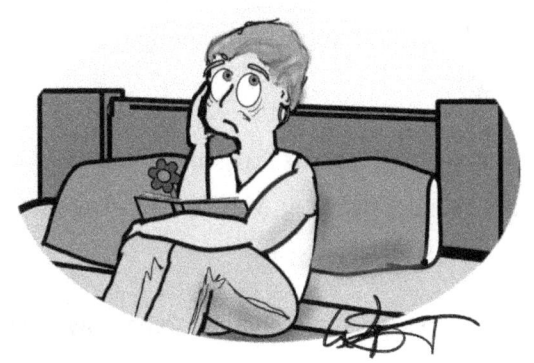

Belle's Diary Entry 4

Dear Diary, I'm writing to you from our bedroom, but I'm alone. Jazz and I had it out, and he's in the guest room.

Jazz came home after 7 again today and dinner was destroyed. He appeared sort of somber. He's aspired into top executive roles now, and they do this thing called 360-assessment, which supervisors, peers and subordinates complete to tell him how he's doing and where to improve. Jazz showed me all the green on it, which I assumed was good feedback, and I said, "Way to go, babe! I'm proud of you."

He then asked me what I thought about a comment that went like this: "Jazz is like a quarterback, a really good one." It was a comment repeated by many. I found it hard to judge how he felt about it: good, bad, or indifferent.

Well, that's why we're not in the same room tonight. I agreed he is a good quarterback, and that I felt like he was calling the plays in our lives as well. I said it's okay to be CEO at work, but at home you still need to do the dishes, dear. I wonder if at work you are directing similarly, and people feel stifled by your brilliance?

That did not land well. He was hurt and swung back with, "Why don't you get some initiative? Maybe then I wouldn't have to always drive."

I didn't like that. It's the reason we're apart now. I was truthful, and he knows it.

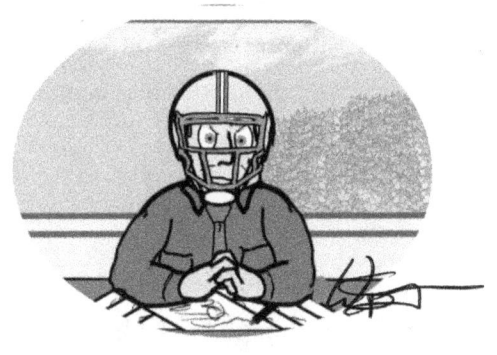

12

Quarterbacking

Luke and Nabal

Hebrews 10:24: "Spur one another on to love and good deeds."

Pearl: "Problems lure egos into solve them."

Luke

I wondered how Nabal was doing after the shooting. I gave him a call to check in.

"Nabal here."

I said, "Hello friend. How are things going?"

"Oh, it is a process of healing. Thank you for asking. It's important to me to keep pushing on. Staff and community—RHS to the rescue—you know the drill. We're focused on a few events to help people recognize mourning and then dancing going forward."

"That's good to do for sure. Anything else?"

Nabal answered, "You are such a good coach and mentor. You get me. Yes, there's something. I think I have an inner saboteur."

I was intrigued. "Hmm, that sounds interesting. If it's an inner one, then you are in control of it?"

"Sort of. Due to all the things we're not supposed to talk about, I was directed to complete a leadership 360-assessment. I've got the results. It's confusing to me."

"How so?" I asked.

"Well, there's a lot of good green rankings," he said. "The assessment says I create a psychological safe workplace, people feel safe, people respect the executive team and me and support them. Yet, from all levels, I got a repetitive comment. It struck me inside. Kind of hit a nerve, man."

"Oh?"

Nabal replied, "Yes. Several comments verbatim were: *Nabal is a good quarterback*. I don't know HOW to take that in the presence of all that is going on. There are lawsuits against me. I got pulled out of my position at one point, then returned to my position as CEO, and now the shooting. I'm perplexed why

QUARTERBACKING

the board has a bullseye on me. I meet with my team members individually and as a group. We have lunches. You know, they say the way to a man's heart is through his stomach. Well, I've adopted that with staff. It seems when we're enjoying a meal, I can get the truth out of people. I drove a strong incident command and now we're healing together. What do you think about that quarterback wording? Is there something in there for me? Is it critical or positive?"

"Language can be a funny thing," I said. "Quarterback, I'm curious how you see a good quarterback? I know you're dealing with stuff. Do you have time to explore this together quickly, or do you want a rain check?"

Nabal said, "That is so like you to put that back on my plate. I get it. I'm good, and it is bugging me, but I'm not sure why. I think of someone who fills an important role on a team. The quarterback touches the ball on every offensive play and so does the center. Plays are critical to the success of a team, and the quarterback usually calls those, like directing and controlling, while leading the team down the field."

I asked him, "Do you find that descriptive of yourself or the assessment feedback?"

"I'm driven. I'm goal-oriented and results matter to me. I delegate a lot. I'm direct but effective," Nabal said. "I have a way of getting to the truth of the matter in my lunch get-togethers. My dad was a pastor. He was strict and had standards. I do too. I feel someone is always watching me. Naomi, my wife, says I never give in. I don't know..."

"Expand on that delegating," I said. "What about your boardroom? What's that like for you and your team?"

Nabal

I sit at the head of the long table because I can see everyone. Here's an example of my frustration. Just today, we had a finding shared from a safety rounding in the in-patient psych ward, which identified that tamper-proof screws were not used in many outlets. We had a close call—a suicide attempt using a rusty screw. Our QM and police chief notified me this morning. It's crazy, but the priority was on the tamper-proof screws, versus the close call. I don't get that. It doesn't fit with my values.

I asked leaders about the finding and their thoughts. Nothing, silence, crickets. I think there was even a full moon! Nothing. Heads were down and it was gloomily quiet. So, as always, I had to pull teeth to get some thoughts and action from the group. Then I asked, "Do we know why this happened?" Still no responses.

I started going down my list I made when I was first notified. I jotted down a few key stakeholders to organize what I thought our next actions should be with his help. As I went through the list of who would do what and completion dates, everyone finally went directly into note-taking mode, following my lead. Heads were nodding and conversations started between them, with some finger-pointing emerging.

I said things like: "Maintenance, you're going to need a team to address this. Do you have a full count of how many? And how soon do you estimate they can be replaced?" "Supply, you'll need to ensure we have enough, and please work with maintenance." "Nursing, please inform the staff of the potential dangers and to be observant. You should work with safety and education." The list went like that. I felt the plan was finally developing; but yeah, I was calling the plays. I guess like a quarterback.

Luke

I asked Nabal, "How do you think that melds into your comments on the assessment?"

"Every time something needs action, I hear this voice in my head telling me that I must drive, because they don't! So, I must. Right? It's my responsibility to make sure actions are taken."

"So, you're feeling responsibility to determine how it is done? Whose voice is that you are hearing?" I asked.

Nabal answered, "My own? It's like I have this sabotage moment that we will fail if I don't take charge. I'm starting to think that my saboteur inner bully crawls out of my words like Freddy Krueger and scares them from speaking up. Is quarterbacking wrong as a CEO?"

"Hey, there's nothing wrong with confident leadership. There are optimal practices and language we can choose to use or not," I answered. "Maybe your choices would benefit from exploration? What comes to your mind about how you might explore? What about these lunches?"

"That is great stuff. I could write down how I give orders or requests and look at softening my language."

"That's an idea worth a journey. When will you do it by? Words matter," I said. "One last observation. You used 'how' versus 'who' and 'why' in your last statement. Does that sound different?"

Nabal responded, "Give me a week? Yes, the word 'how' opens my mind to possibilities. My words are closed. My questions direct because I can't get anywhere unless I dig, and dig deep. They will only talk when alone. It seems they prefer this group talk. They even had a meeting I was not invited to. They say it is to be sure they are solving things at the lowest possible level."

"Hmmm..."

"I also wonder if asking 'why' turned out to be a bit too sharp and accusatory? I might have put more blame in the room, simply by my words. Wow, I knew you would be helpful to get me into my mind. I'm going to try using the word 'how' to give them the freedom to think and speak. I'm also going to empower my team to see the end of the field the way they see it, versus driving them down to my touchdown."

I said, "Deal. See you at the big corporate meeting! Your resilience paid off for your team and community, buddy. You are a lot of folks' hero! Keep on keeping on. Hey, if you don't already, might I suggest you journal your thoughts, so next time we talk, you can recall all the details of things and your insights?"

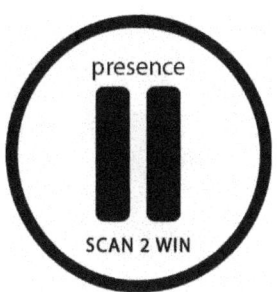

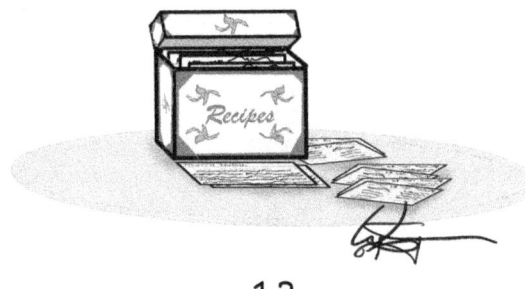

13

Burgers, Babble, and the Last Supper

```
Nabal and Naomi
```

Proverbs 16:28 "Perverse people stir conflict; a gossip separates friends."

Pearl: "Keep friends close and enemies closer."

Nabal

"Naomi, how about you meet me for lunch today at the hospital? I know how you love Berger's Burgers, our new hospital café."

"Sure, Nabal, that sounds fun. I am excited about getting a strawberry shake. I'd like to talk to you about how to redecorate our great room."

"Oh, good. I have some ideas about that too. Why would you want a strawberry shake when they have such amazing malts? You do you, girl. See you at noon?"

Naomi

My heart was racing, pounding, and almost stopped. A disruptive voice came from deep inside me saying, *Nabal is not like that. He loves me. Mean is what Mom did to me. I still can't take a bath because she made me sleep in that bathtub when she was entertaining men. He's not like that. He loves me. My college fling wouldn't let me even get in the same room as other guys... so controlling and suspicious. I still remember the date when he spilled that chocolate malt on my new white sundress just to embarrass me in front of a football player. He's not like that, either. He loves me. Do I need to run away again like I did when I was 17? Nah, he's not like that. He loves me.*

Nabal

I thought to myself, *I guess Luke was on to something. I'll journal this frustration I'm feeling.*

Dear Journal, I don't know how to fix this team. I've asked God for help. A chaplain comes to my office weekly, and we pray about life, and the organization, and for all of them, too. I am open about my core beliefs. Maybe that's an issue offending them. Christ did say that if they despise and hated Him, they will hate me too.

BURGERS, BABBLE, AND THE LAST SUPPER

I'm not the best man in the world, that's for sure. I am different because of this place. Today was no exception. It was another exasperating meeting with these people. I don't even have time to think about Naomi anymore. They are like an impenetrable wall at times. The only way I can get anywhere with them is to get them individually alone with me and give them food. Divide and conquer. They talk only then and are so friendly. They become quite open-minded and, in some cases, even agreeable over a burger and a malt. This morning's meeting went nowhere. We really need to get our safety improved for patients in our mental health units. I'm worried that we're going to have a terrible thing happen soon.

Is Naomi ok? She seems like she wants to do something.

I spoke with the engineering department and the COO today. It was nothing less than stonewalling, and they were pretty good at making me feel pushy and not strategic. They said they would change priorities and do the remodeling of the mental health unit first, but when the summer came, there were unprecedented heat complaints from staff of the failed air conditioning system. "It will be like a furnace in the C-suite, boss." Even the head nurse was against the realignment of priorities because of her health concerns due to the heat. Naomi mentioned our AC at home was a bit wonky. I don't have time for that now. We'll call someone.

What do I need to do to get a mission and vision in here? When do we talk about patients? Well, Dr. Luke, we'll see what you have in your wisdom well for this one. I'm stuck. Wow, it's 12:15. I'm late. *Journal entry end.*

My mind was still going as I rushed to the restaurant. There was Naomi, sitting in a booth, waiting on me. Pretty common for me to be undependable. I apologized for being late. Did I even say hi or give her a kiss? I don't know. She was understanding. It sure seemed she had some personal agenda to go over with me, too. Why is it that when these things come up something always needs fixed or correcting by me? I don't know how much more of this I can take. Everyone wants their way, even Naomi. What about the mission? What about me? Why doesn't anyone care but me? Can she hear me?

I started right out of the blue, with no regard for her or lunch. "Naomi, I think I really struck a nerve with them today. I asked them to cancel their private morning meeting, and they agreed they didn't need it and could use the time in their calendars. I thought that was a win for fresh communication. Maybe we're getting somewhere. Should we order?"

Naomi looked like a deer in the headlights but said yeah. I kept thinking, *what if they lied and held the meeting secretly?* They still have the same dialogue and responses. They're always sheepishly deceptive, yet willing to do whatever I say in their words. Yet, their execution of the deed is another story. Is that the quarterback thing?

They're like that old article from the 1970s, "Swimming with Sharks." I think I may either be in bloody waters or I'm wounded and bleeding. This is attracting the sharks to me. That article says to get out of the water or hit them on the nose. I think I've tried both. What does a quarterback do when the team is either huddling in the locker room or just stuck to the bench? How do

BURGERS, BABBLE, AND THE LAST SUPPER

I show them the end zone? What I need is a gin and tonic or Valium.

Naomi was saying something. I felt dizzy. "Uh, Nabal, are we going to order?" Naomi's voice broke through my brain fog. We ordered. I got a malt, and she ordered her strawberry shake.

She began, "I was thinking we should lighten up the furniture to a cream color and get some new artwork for the great room."

I said, "Well, not only that, but we also really need to start with pulling up the wood floor. It's a disaster of scratches. We need a new floor first. Why would we want to put lipstick on a pig versus getting the pig a manicure?"

Naomi had a look of dejection. I knew then I was in for it.

She then said, "Listen, I have ideas. You can't own everyone and everything. Sometimes, others do have thoughts. Were you insinuating that our home is a pig? I keep the house clean, do your laundry, pick up after you and all I ask is a little freedom to dream and make our nest a home. You can leave your dirty underwear on your new floor, and I won't be there to care. How would you like that?"

I should have kept my mouth shut and my thoughts to myself, but I retorted quietly so no one would overhear us. "Naomi, you can do you. If you like missing out on a fabulous malt or settling for a strawberry shake, that's all on you. I'm going to do me. I've got crazy people working here that I can't get through to, nor can I trust. You know they call me a quarterback. I don't even feel like second-string in this place most days."

Naomi struck back. "You might be a quarterback, but you're not going to the Superbowl with me either, mister."

My phone went off. "Naomi, we can discuss this later. I'm sorry for being short. Maybe lunch here was not my best idea. I do a lot of business meetings here and I was not all with you. I've got to run. They need me upstairs. Rain check? I'll see you at home. Enjoy your burger, and I know, you love the strawberry. I'm going to make it up to you. I promise."

Naomi

Well, he's gone again, like a fancy suit gone in a flash. Just like when my old boss used to buzz through our cubicle area, saying, "Is everyone doing good?" We'd all say yes and off she'd jet to her office, close the door, and repeat it at the end of the shift. We'd all go home feeling like she wasn't even there.

He wasn't here with me. Nope, not at all. He didn't even listen to my ideas. He was too caught up in thinking about his next words. Here I sit in that bathtub alone again, like I messed up a blind date or something. This is not a bathtub, it's a booth. Am I wrong to want just a little something of my personal mark on things? No, I'm not wrong. He's wrong.

He's under so much pressure. Nabal loves me. He's not like Mom and the others. I wish I could just strangle some of these people that should be respectful and work with him. If he treats them the way he just treated me, oh boy, is he in for an awakening. I know they're bad, but his choices aren't helping the matter.

BURGERS, BABBLE, AND THE LAST SUPPER

Nabal says he's always alone. I know what being alone is, buddy. I don't know who this man is any more or what he is thinking.

I wish Nabal was here now. We do need a new floor, but couldn't we at least get artwork? I'm so mad at him, but I miss him.

Four important people sat down at a table across from me. I wondered if it could be his terrorist team. Two men and two women. In between bites of my burger and slurps of my shake, I was enthralled by their interactions. They looked angry yet determined.

The first guy (COO) said, "What a relief to be away from that self-righteous tyrant." The talk went on from there. Quite an interesting dialogue it became.

The second guy (Chief Plant Operations) said, "Yes, I don't know what we're going to do. He really wants us to burn the place down, literally. Who does he think he is? God? Why does all the staff seem to love this character? What has he done to our simple life and hospital?"

A woman (CNO) said, "I can't deal with the heat again. Mental health is not going to melt. We will. Why do we have to keep going through the same things over and over?"

The first man said, "Can you believe he told us to stop meeting as a team? What a control freak. He asks so many questions it is daunting and keeping me from my work. I feel judged every time I'm around him. He's exactly the type of church Bible banger my dad warned me about. My schedule is unpredictable, and

I can't keep answering his spontaneous beckoning. Don't you dread when he invites you here? It's sermon time."

A second woman, the CFO, said, "I don't know if he's a freak. It's just he's new. We've had so many interim CEOs. Shouldn't we give him a chance? A bit more time? Let's just sit him down and tell him how we're feeling."

The first woman said, "Are you kidding me? We all decided on this a month ago. Today was my last straw. He's got to go. I will just make sure the nurses are watching for these stupid little screws. It's not that big of a deal to me. Unbelievable, this is what he puts priority on—it wasn't a completed suicide. It was just an attempt. These patients cry out like this in that unit quite all the time. It's part of their illness. We got this. We're professional care providers. He sure can't see what's important in healthcare. I am feeling crucified by him."

The second woman responded, "I suppose so. The last time he spoke with me, he told me that all of you told him individually you questioned my effectiveness as a leader. Is that true?"

The first man answered, "Absolutely not. There's no way I'm diverting plans we've had for years just because he's a nervous nellie about these screws. I sure didn't say that about you or your leadership. You always make sure my budget is on track. So, when I get my money, I am happy."

"Hey, isn't it kind of funny we're meeting here at the same burger joint?" the second man asked. "He sure likes to bring us here and drill us like water boarding torture. This is his last supper, I hope. Can you believe the Bible verses on his desk? Courageous? Strong? Should say 'wife beater'!"

The first woman added, "For certain. Last time I was here for 'lunch' with the creep, he talked about you and how he doesn't understand your reluctance to do the minor repairs to mental health. He wanted to know what I thought you were thinking when you say no to him. I'm like, I'm no psychologist or mind reader. It was weird. I just shrugged. Then later in the day, his assistant came in and asked me the same question. As if I'm going to tell her anything. You know, we should have fired her a long time ago. She's also a big problem here; getting into everyone's business and the gossip is ridiculous."

The first man said, "Well, if all of you would have supported me just a little more during the last round of CEO hiring, I wouldn't be number two, having to do number one's job. We might not be here devising a plan today to rid ourselves of yet another misfit."

"I had a similar experience," said the second woman. "He was digging for dirt on you too, honey. He wanted to know why nurses weren't working with the ED from the floors. I told him I'm an accountant, sir. He said, 'Well, we're all a team, right?' I can't believe the nerve of this guy. He is an outsider. We were doing just fine before he showed up."

The first man said, "So, we don't have a lot of time. I spoke with our HR friend. She said we should file four individual complaints, and that it would be strong if we had some of our line chiefs send in similar complaints. She told me the board would wait on the reports. We can get rid of this idiot and go on doing what we do best—running this hospital. This time vote me in as CEO."

The second man said, "You've got my support, sir. Show me the money! Uh... by the way, I might have an idea how we can pressure influence on the general staff to get them to turn on him."

"What you got stewing?" asked the first man.

The second man answered, "Well, you know how we all have our pictures on the first floor. You remember a couple years ago when staff keyed the old nurse's car and put sticky notes on his picture? That sent him to the hills. Maybe it will work again."

"That's ingenious," said the first man. "How will you pull it off?"

The second man responded, "Give me a day or two. I'll get it done, sir. Remember, the police chief owes me a favor. We'll get him wanting to leave for fear alone. In fact, I'm just going to set the maintenance team on the air conditioning repair today. It will be done by the end of the week. We'll get to mental health when I feel like it fits."

The first woman chimed in, "Ugh, anything is better than him staying. I've posted my resume already, just because I can't stand change, or him. Maybe there's hope I can stay here."

I walked over there to see what that was all about. I probably shouldn't have, but if this was Nabal they were discussing, I'm his wife. I didn't like this. "Excuse me, you all look quite important. Might I ask where the patient advocates' office is located?"

BURGERS, BABBLE, AND THE LAST SUPPER

The second woman asked me, "Do you have a problem?"

I responded, "I couldn't help but overhearing your conversation and it struck me as your culture here is struggling. I want to be sure that my healthcare isn't equally struggling. You seem not happy and I'm sorry, but this type of conversation probably shouldn't be happening where a patient like me can overhear you. What are your thoughts on that?"

The woman said, "I'm sorry. Who are you? What is your concern? Our hospital has some of the best metrics in the region. Is there something we can do for you?"

"I'm Nabal's wife. That's who I am. I'm heading to the spa because you all stressed me out. You should be ashamed."

Nabal

I thought to myself, *I need to make this up to Naomi. She's my only friend and person I can trust. I'm going to call that art gallery and get the designer out to the house tonight. Yeah, I'll surprise her. She can buy all the art she wants then. Plus, I will just call the furniture store and have them deliver the cream set. Yeah, that way she will see I am attentive and care. I just don't know how much more of this I can take. I still have time to get this done before she gets home from her spa day.*

Back at home, the furniture looked amazing, and the designer was there, just as Naomi pulled into the garage. I couldn't wait to surprise her.

Naomi entered. "Hello, Nabal. How was your day?"

I said, "Like any other, except I hurt my best friend, and I'm sorry. I've done some things to make your day better. Come on inside, dear."

Naomi's eyes were wide and full of welled-up tears. She recognized the designer and said hello. I grabbed her a Kleenex and hugged her. I said, "I thought about our conversation earlier and why I'm hanging us up in suspense about the furniture. So, I had it delivered. Do you love it?"

Naomi said, "I do. I wanted one last look, but yes, this was sweet of you to take control once again and get it done."

Our designer was there to help us get just the right art. I had not called a contractor about the floor just yet. Thought maybe the art might change things.

It was a good evening, but I could tell something was eating at her. Still, she was resilient through it all. The designer left, and we sat on the new sofa in a strange quiet. Naomi got up and put some laundry in the washer, then came and sat in front of me on the ottoman. I sensed she had just been through the entire spin cycle of a washing machine. She looked rough. I was feeling rough.

She opened with, "Nabal, I met your team today."

Naomi

They were in the burger joint and sat at a table. They were discussing you. They were ugly. You're right. They are out to get you. I'm scared now that we have new furniture and expensive

BURGERS, BABBLE, AND THE LAST SUPPER

art. What if they succeed? Nabal, I don't know how you can deal with this. I worry that our relationship at home has deteriorated. We're at each other a lot lately. It's not like you.

They said nasty things about how you take them to the restaurant and interrogate them. Sometimes, dearest husband, I feel the same. So, for a moment there, I was identifying with the terrorist group. They don't know your heart like I do. I love you. I support you. I am asking you to please get help.

I will tell you that your nurse is rude, obnoxious, prideful, and dismissive of others, including me. I asked where the patient advocate was located, and all she could do was insinuate if I had a problem or concern, it was mine. She rattled off some statistics, and well, then she got frustrated and asked who I was and what I wanted.

Nabal

I thought, *Oh my God. My sweet Jesus.* "Honey, I need some time. Just a second or two to process all of this. I am so sorry you met them. Yes, I have changed. I must."

I told Naomi how I'd had to go back to my office just after the furniture was delivered, and when I walked by my photograph, it was vandalized. It said things about my salary and my demeanor. It was ugly. I called the police to investigate it. They took pictures, and I came home. What an emotional day for both of us.

I believe that those people on my team had something to do with that threatening message. It's funny because just a day or so ago, I was speaking with the plant chief, and he told me the previous interim CEO and nurse had some vandalism to their cars and pictures were obliterated with a Sharpie.

Naomi said, "I would agree. They were devising a plan when I overheard them. It sounded like one of them wants your job and has applied for it several times. Do you trust the police to find this out, or do you want me to do a report of what I heard?"

I said, "Unfortunately, they all have worked together for several years. I doubt your report would help. I'll let the police do their thing. If it makes you feel better, go ahead and do an anonymous report."

Naomi said, "I shall. I do love the furniture. For our next purchase, could we do it together? I'd really like to be a couple again. I want to know that you want to do this for me."

I pulled Naomi in close and kissed her forehead. That reminded me of something I heard in church once: *"Keep your enemies closer than a friend."*

I slept in just a bit more today. Naomi said she had an early start. I walked into the kitchen to have a cup of coffee and spilled it on my feet, burning through my socks. I could not believe my eyes. My worst nightmare happened. There on the counter by the Keurig, was a disarray of recipe cards, but two had Naomi's writing on them.

I read:

BURGERS, BABBLE, AND THE LAST SUPPER 191

Dearest Nabal, I know this is going to be tough. I just can't keep doing this with you. The pressure is too much. My stomach is a mess, and I can't sleep. It reminds me of my abusive mom and a college boyfriend. My mom locked me in the bathroom, and I had to sleep alone in the tub. She had lots of men over and didn't want me getting in the way of her fun. Mom did this often and for no reason. She said it bought me nice clothes. She was thinking only of herself.

My longest relationship besides you was with a college man who controlled my every move. He even threw a shake at me once, to mess up my dress in public. He wouldn't let me talk to any other guys. I never told you any of this because I see a bit of him in you. The minute I turned 17, I ran away and never looked back. You know I don't talk about my mom, and we have never gone to visit. I fell madly in love with you. I thought you were different. Thank you for not locking me up, but you have locked me out of your heart, and your words do matter. I feel controlled again.

The times when you don't include or interrogate me bring this memory, and I don't like how I had to cower and submit. I don't like how I feel now. There are issues in all our lives, my sweetest. You have yours and I have mine. I refuse to freeze like a shake or malt, no matter what your microaggressions are. Ridiculous, Nabal!

Yesterday, I nearly said that to you about the shake/malt comments you made. It hurt and convinced me we need space if we're prioritizing trivial things. Then I hear this awful talk from people who you lead. You need space. Please ask for help. Don't be proud to lose our marriage, friendship or what we may have. It's too late for me. I just don't know. I can't take anymore. My mother is ill and needs me. I don't want to go there, but it seems like the right thing to do. I need a change and time.

I'm calling a lawyer and pastor to see what is next in my life. You will be fine. You'll see. Please don't call me. Maybe in a couple of weeks when I've had time to clear my head. I'm sorry these are on recipe cards. I didn't want to wake you. Love, Naomi.

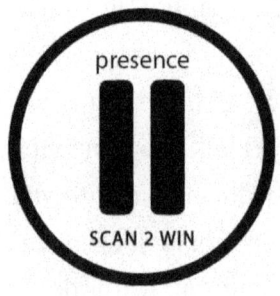

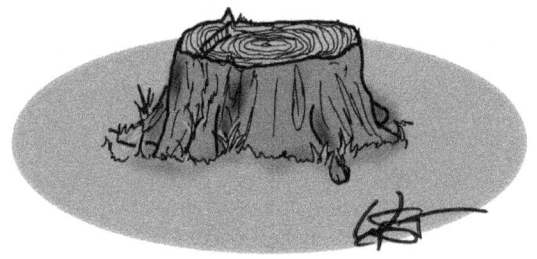

Belle's Diary Entry 5

What's Over There?

Today I asked Jazz to go for a walk. He was reluctant, but he did. He's gone from playing with his dinner to just sitting and staring. Jazz will pace for like 15 minutes or so, then just plop into a chair and stare. Once I turned the TV up so loud it hurt my ears, yet it didn't faze him. I wondered what was over there where he was staring.

I sat next to him today and rubbed his back. He pulled away and looked at me with steel in his eyes. He said, "Why did you do that?"

I went to the kitchen. "Nope, not going to let it end like this again. Jazz, let's go for that walk now."

"Now?" he asked.

"Yes, now. Get up and let's go."

We did. It was midday and sunny. I asked him what he was staring at. He stopped, and we sat on a stump together. Jazz opened his heart and finally spoke about it. He told me he felt like a failure, and that there was nothing else he could do to lead people who didn't want to be part of a team. Then he told me he felt he had failed me and our love. He said he remembered the day we met and wished we could go back to those easier days. Jazz said he didn't want to work anymore, and some of his trusted colleagues told him he was not well. He asked my opinion.

I said, "I think you could use a pause, maybe."

He said, "I quit today. I just walked out, and I am on family medical leave. Let's just move back to the UP."

At first, I was scared to death, but I had my Jazz back in my arms. He was no longer tied to whatever was over there he was staring at. So, I asked him again, "Jazz, what's over where you were staring?"

He said, "It's a Humvee crashing towards me and you. It's going to take us out. There's no way I can protect you from it unless I quit. I won't give up trying unless I just say goodbye. It's a heart attack or cancer or something else gruesome. I see darkness and no hope over there."

I asked him, "Why do you stare at it, honey?"

He said, "It makes me curious about what my life, our life, is all about. I think God has more for us to do and we are imprisoned here. He put us here. No question. But we're being called now, and God is making it fully apparent to me. I'm afraid of giving all this up, like the rich young ruler in the Bible. It must be done. Do you agree?"

I said, "Yes, Jazz. Let's go home and go with God."

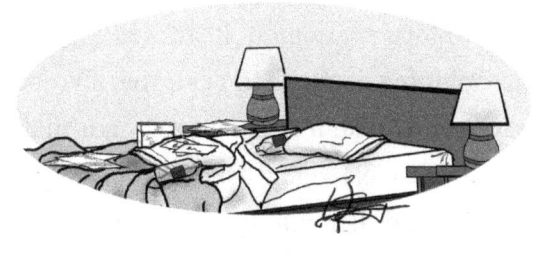

14

Gathering Grief

Ezekiel's Journal

Hebrews 10:25 "Meet with one another."

Pearl: "Change your lens often to keep from blurring."

There are times in life when you just must journal it. There are fears and triumphs that I must write down to see later and make a withdrawal from that bank of wisdom and hard knocks. This is one of those.

The flight was long, and I was tired. I just wanted to get through the hotel lobby and to my room. I thanked the shuttle driver and approached the doorways. I dreaded dragging two suitcases, a briefcase, and the bulky computer case through revolving doors. Plus, I cheated on my diet and had the driver swing in that familiar drive thru.

Not a big fan of escalators in airports, either. I avoid it, and of course, the other door was marked with that yellow wet floor sign. So, I had to face my demon. It seemed this time this evil creature was spinning faster than any other I've been in. My extra suitcase seemed like it had a magnet in it that intuitively stuck to the metal frame, lodging itself in front of me. It clunked and wound up ejected right into the lobby!

Once inside, there was Nabal, picking up my bag, laughing. It was funny and embarrassing. Nabal said, "It's good to see you finally. We've got a lot to talk about."

I agreed and expressed how tonight I needed to make an early evening of it. I said, "Let's hook up tomorrow." I checked in and snuck up to my room. I think Nabal was drinking some. He smelled. Called Miriam, said our nightly I love you, ate my ninety-nine-cent heart attack bag meal and shrugged off my shortness of breath and racing pulse. I brushed my teeth, ran an iron over my suit and slipped into the sheets. Just a couple hours later, I woke up to the obnoxious buzzing of the hotel clock-radio/alarm. The previous guest must have had a red-eye flight, and I forgot to unplug it. I always unplug it. I heard myself saying, "Why didn't you do that this time, dummy?!" I turned over, pulled the pillow on my head, and finally fell asleep.

What a night. I was dressed and headed to the meeting room. There I found all my colleagues. Nabal and Luke were at the head table because they're big shots now. I sat in the back with my good bud, Esther. At least 200 people were here this time. It was awesome to see them all. The RHS Corporate Office was all here. Last time I saw them was online during COVID. Wonder if there will be a big announcement? We were supposed to be updated about a raise for all of us and our staff. Well, it was rumored, as well as a possible new acquisition.

The first item addressed was the mass shooting in Nabal's city. The corporate leaders acknowledged what strong leadership and culture Nabal drove. They said his resilience made all the difference. We shared a moment of silence, and the corporate chaplain led us in a remembrance. It was nice and needed. Nabal stood at the podium and debriefed the horrible event, and his lessons learned. We all took copious notes. We applauded as Nabal took it in. He seemed distant, yet there. Then, we moved on with the standard agenda. There were various speakers and power points. Oh, the death by power point for hours.

We broke for lunch.

It is welded in my neurons. Last night Nabal was so gracious to help me with that runaway bag, as I sheepishly sought sleep and sanctuary, postponing our chill time together. How could anyone ever had predicted what would be next?

We reassembled from lunch for the afternoon sessions. These sessions focused on lowering our contract care reliance. I and others were deeply attentive and engaged in fixing our bottom line. Lots of emotions and barriers were shared, as well as some creative success stories. During the last break, I noticed Nabal wasn't in the break area. I texted. Nothing. I thought, *Heck, this is a longer break. I'm going to take a walk.*

My walk led me past Nabal's room, where I found the door just a bit ajar and a laundry cart with disorganized linen parked next to it. I knocked. Nothing. I texted again. Nothing. I knocked. Nothing. My deepest intuition twinged. Something was up. I knocked. I pushed the door slightly, to confirm that it was truly ajar, and said, "Hello, Nabal. You here?" Nothing. Again, my intuition pushed me deeper into the room.

The bedroom suite door was slightly open, and I saw 3 envelopes neatly placed at the end of the bed on a single pillow. The rest of the room was a disaster. It was tussled like a couple of wrestlers had a championship match in it. There were papers and empty gin bottles strewn all over it and on the floor. There also was a small metal box that looked like a recipe card box. The papers appeared to be depositions and notification letters. I ignored the three envelopes and walked with uncertain trepidation towards the bathroom door. I pushed on it just as the housekeeper entered behind me.

It was simultaneous.

The door slid open easily. I sank, and the housekeeper screamed.

I had found Nabal.

He was hanging from the shower door with a sheet wrapped around his neck and several towels neatly placed on the floor beneath him. He was not breathing and had no heartbeat.

That's when I dialed 911. The housekeeper just vanished. I fell to my knees. I felt like I was stuck in that revolving door and could not get out. My worst fears had replicated. My God, how could this... why did he... when did he... what could be so bad? All those terrible questions were yelling inside me. All the bad history. What will his family do? The paramedics were not far behind, but it was truly too late. He was gone.

News somehow got to the corporate leaders, and two of them appeared shortly afterward in the hallway outside. They were so respectful and professional, yet I sensed they too shared my deep astonishment and pain. They informed me the meeting was adjourned, and we'd resume in the morning. They offered me help and encouraged me to seek it, as this was a tragedy and trauma. No one asked me why I was there. I appreciated that. They said there was an announcement of an "untimely death."

I don't know why, but I took all three envelopes. Maybe because the top one had my name on it. After sifting through them, I discovered another for Nabal's wife's name, Naomi, and the last letter was addressed to God. Lofting in the air was a pungent odor, reminiscent of my son's bedroom and apartment of gin. It hurt and scared me.

The last time we talked was over a year ago. All the late-night visits to the sheriff's office to bail him out of the drunk tank. I couldn't go to my room. I could barely walk. I couldn't think. I couldn't even feel. I called Miriam, and we sobbed together while I walked. I ran out of breath several times as we prayed for Nabal, his family, and Abel.

She is so good to me. She said, "Are you okay? You'd better call Sage. Don't you think? He's good for you."

I thought about it for a nanosecond and lied. "Yeah, I'm good. (to protect her) And yes, I'll call him."

As she gently ended the call, I wound up right back in that spinning doorway, just like my ejected suitcase that flew into the lobby of hell. It wasn't the kind of doorway or escalator that got me—it was my return from Iraq. From every direction, it flooded into me. I flashed back to the sandpit. We lost many soldiers in fighting and even friendly fire. But it was the suicides that were especially impactful upon me when I got back home. Several times I had to discipline soldiers for multiple Driving While Intoxicated charges. One took his life, and the scene was just like this one.

This was the reason I left the Army after years of success. I just couldn't prevent it from happening. I couldn't fix it. I couldn't fix them. I can't fix my son. I had to tell so many people this type of news, and it dug deep into me. At times, I cannot be in a large room alone because I am reminded of my command office and preparations for those awful rides to family homes. Sometimes I carried the note to the family. It was my darkest and most sad place. Yet here I am again.

I had hoped this new role in healthcare would not subject me to it ever again, let alone today. I thought about that darned hotel alarm. Why didn't I hear Nabal's alarm? I should have done something. I didn't see a clue that he needed me or anyone. He was laughing. Why this letter to me? Why not someone else he knew? I trembled to open it. How could I rank among his wife and family? How does one deliver a letter to God? Why me? Why me?

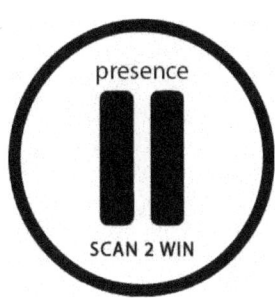

PRESENCE PAUSE: *This presence pause is much different. I've added some questions due to the content and graphic nature of the story.*

Please ask yourself:

How am I right now in this moment?

Were there any memories or triggers for me?

Do I need to speak with someone?

Please dial 988 if you do.

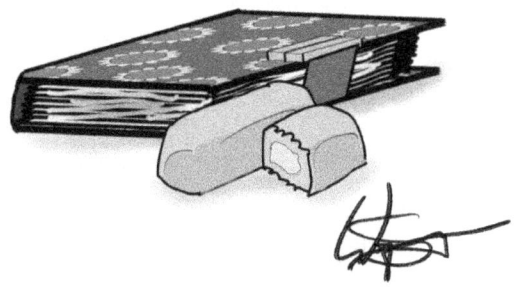

15

Going Through the Hoops

Miriam and Sarah's Phone Call

Hebrews 10:25 "Meet with one another."

Pearl: "Don't eat the cheese or take the Twinkie."

Miriam

It was a grand spring morning. Ezekiel was off at his office catching up, or so he said. He'd sure been at the office a lot lately since that tragic loss of Nabal. I relaxed in our favorite chairs by the picture window, watching the cardinals at the feeders. I remember my mother telling me, "Where there are cardinals, there are angels nearby."

My phone rang. "Hello?"

"Hello, Miriam?"

"Yes?"

"This is Sarah, Sage's wife. How are you, dear? I often think of our ski trip, and just came across your number in my sweater pocket. I thought, well there's a sign I should call the girl and see what you've been up to. Plus, I just need a friendly ear."

"Oh my, Sarah, I think we are birds of a feather. We're doing well. Ezekiel is working late a lot and on the weekends. Here it is Sunday, and we didn't go to church. Instead, we had a devotion, and he popped off with his briefcase in shorts and a ball cap to the office. I was just admiring our cardinals at the backyard feeder."

Sarah interrupted. "Oh, yes, and those are little angel signs, you know!"

"Yes, in fact, you read my mind. We really do have a nice connection, you and me. I'm so glad you called, because I was feeling a bit down. I suppose Sage and Ezekiel have each other. Why not us?"

"Yes, dear, why not us?"

"What's on your mind, Sarah?"

Sarah

Well, you're going to think I'm just a silly worry wort of a grandma. My daughter and I are quite close, and she lives only a few miles from us, so it is nice we get to see the granddaughters often. My, how they grow, and cute as a button! It's been a couple months now that our oldest, Isabella, who is six and in kindergarten, has become much different and it is concerning me. She gives the grandest hugs and is so very thoughtful. She often will go up to strangers and just strike up a conversation about a hat they might be wearing. At the grocer, she always brings a smile to the cashier. She's just been a doll to enjoy growing up. But recently she has become, well, the darned old serpent himself!

She is defiant and will challenge her mother and me on just about anything. Not getting to bed on time, being a sloth on the way to school. Yesterday, my daughter and I took Isabella out on a date, and for no reason at all, she just ran off in a mall. I am old and slow and couldn't keep up. When I did get an eye on her, she refused to come to me, and I lost track of her again. My goodness, my heart was pounding, and thoughts were racing because you know how bad people steal children these days and do the most awful things to humans.

We caught her when she ran right into the store security officer's knees. A perfect lesson. Nope. She told him, "You can't arrest me, mister. I'm just a little girl." Oh, her mom and I let her know how dangerous it was. She just smirked at us, as if she wanted the angry attention. We firmly planted her cuteness in a shopping cart the rest of the time at the mall and then went home. It's interesting, however, at her school conferences the teachers all say she's the good little girl we used to see and more! They say she's a leader and sets examples for others. We're in a stew here.

I recall you saying you all have a grown son. Does he have children? I don't remember if you two had arrived at the silver honor state of grandparenthood.

Miriam

"No, not yet," I replied. "He struggles with his own demons, and we are there with him, or at least we try. It is very tough when alcohol clouds a person's true authenticity and kindness. That is what happens with Abel. We haven't spoken in quite some time."

Sarah said, "I can only imagine. We're never given more than we can handle, I suppose."

I agreed.

Sarah

So, two weeks ago, our daughter was fed up with the Girl Scout leader and the troop. Well, I wouldn't even call this a troop. There are only 4 little ones in the group.

The leader is younger, and focused on selling cookies, getting badges, and competing with the larger, established troops in the nearby cities. This troop never says the Girl Scout pledge or the Pledge of Allegiance. There's no way they can keep up. She's gone to the point of segregating the kindergartners from the first graders because her daughter is a first grader. Our little Isabella is being discriminated against in Girl Scouts! It got to a point where the leader's daughter, a first grader, has taken it upon herself and another first grader to tease and bully innocent Isabella.

They say things like, "Why is your hair such a mess? Why can't you color like a first grader? Your mommy doesn't love you." It's just unforgiveable. Kids can be so mean and unthoughtful. I blame the parents. That's what I say. Apples don't fall far, you know.

Our daughter finally had enough and told this leader that Isabella would no longer be in the troop. The leader and another mother are now bullying our daughter by calling and leaving messages about what is going on and things they believe our daughter should still do. We all are at the point of turning bully on this leader, and next time telling her something like, "Oh, my. Isabella and our family are picking belly button lint that day and won't be able to sell cookies. Remember, we quit?"

Miriam

We both giggled nervously. I chimed in. "Sarah, that is so funny you'd say this today. Our nephew, the lawyer, has a couple of wonderful boys. One is six—same as Isabella—sweet as they come, but they are noticing changes in him since he has gone to public school and kindergarten. John called yesterday and shared a cute story. He said he, his wife, and their little fella, Mark, were at a fancy dinner. They ordered, and the customary salad and breadsticks were promptly delivered to the table. Mark was plowing through the breadsticks, not eating any salad, and John said to him, 'Mark, no more breadsticks. You'll spoil your dinner.' John said the punchline was delivered by his wife, who asked him if he was planning on eating all four breadsticks on his plate!"

Goose—Gander, they say! Together we chanted: "Kids!"

As we shared about the bullying exploits of our little ones, it brought back a memory of mine. Not proud of it, but I felt I had to get it off my chest.

"Sarah?" I asked. "I have a bullying memory of my own. Can I share?"

"Oh, indeed do, girlfriend!"

I was always a fast runner in middle school track. I won a lot of races, and by a lot of distance between me and the others. I grew up in a small town of about three thousand people. Everyone knew everyone, and all about everyone—that type of quaint Americana. My parents were not well-to-do, and we had a family of seven kids. My mom never had any sugar or junk food in the house. She told us it would rot our teeth, and our brains would fall into paralysis if we ate it!

So, you can guess when I saw junk food, I was envious and wanted to try it. Honestly, I'd never had a Twinkie. I used to ponder that soft yellow cushion of goodness, and how that smooth white cream would glide upon my tongue. Sometimes, I imagined taking it apart slowly and... well, you get the point. I was infatuated with Twinkies.

I had a notebook I kept as a journal of romantic poems and my thoughts. I always had it with me. It looked like a high-class business planner with its golden threaded book marker and latchet. It was flowered with sunflowers and a lush, dark green background. I loved it. It was my heart and deepest thought companion.

There was a girl named Delilah, who was on the track team with me. Delilah was a horribly slow runner, and she was quite mean. Her gift was the shot put, and she was great at hurling that orb. She had this crew of others she ran with, and they would terrorize the rest of us girls, especially my best friend and me. One time she went in the shower and put blue ink all over my friend's towel. When she came out, ink was all over her body and face.

It was never-ending, and we all avoided confrontations with them. I remember my worst Delilah moment was when she grabbed my notebook in class. It was awful, and she promptly began reading a page out loud! It was a note and a poem about a boy I hoped would notice me. Well, Delilah read it all mushy-like and teasing. Then she said, "Scoochie Koo. Miriam will never get a boy like you!" I snatched my notebook and fled the classroom. I was destroyed. The boy knew it was him, and he shook his head and laughed.

Here's the part I'm not too proud of. When I returned to the classroom, I saw Delilah had a TWINKIE, of all things, in her backpack. It was just peeking its little cuteness out of the side pocket, and it appeared reachable. I thought I'd slide it loose from its backpack prison camp and into my loving hands. That would teach her a thing or two.

I could not get that darned Twinkie out of my mind. I had to have it. We had a race that afternoon, so I devised a plan. I caught Delilah in the hall outside after class on the way to the locker room. I beguiled her. "Delilah, I know you haven't run a race and won first place. How would you like it if you did win?" She, of course, was all in. We agreed I would run slower, and she would pass me up and win. All I asked for was, you guessed it, THE TWINKIE!

Delilah looked at me with those steely blue eyes. Then, out of nowhere, came the God of Heaven's voice bellowing from her mouth. "Okay, I win, you get the Twinkie. You really are so shallow. Scoochie Koo, nobody loves you." I couldn't believe it. Then my mind went to how to cover up with my mom if she was at the race. Was the Twinkie going to be a public baton handoff, or would it happen in a dark alley behind the school after midnight? My mind wouldn't stop racing with the possible solutions and outcomes. I was like an addict, a Twinkie addict. I had to have my fix. Would this deal slow Delilah's bullying?

BANG went the starting gun, and off we bolted. I started at my usual speed—fast—and took an early large lead. Then I realized I must lose this race, and Delilah needs to win for me to get my Twinkie prize. I slowed and turned my head back and to the side. Where was Delilah? She was in dead last, trudging along. Was she playing me? I slowed more. I felt like a turtle and must have looked the part. The crowd noticed. I didn't see my mom, so that was good.

People started chanting for me to run faster, but I slowed down like molasses were in my legs. Four girls passed me, then I passed them. Finally, there came Delilah. It was just me and Delilah. The finish line seemed like a mile away, yet it was just the final stretch. I slowed almost to a stop; Delilah passed by. The crowd was chanting my name by then, and well, time ran out. Delilah ran by, and I took second. Delilah won, and it was time for the Twinkie. I had imagined this wonderful reward all along, and how it would feel holding its translucent plastic in my palm at last. I thought of that poem and fate, how we were going to be together. Then, Delilah threw the Twinkie at me and yelled, "Here, Scoochie Koo. Here's your prize. I shouldn't give it to you because you made it so obvious I didn't win, and you threw the race. But here, you deserve it."

I felt diminished by Delilah's verbal abuse, and from my own inner bully telling me how terrible of a person I am. I snuck away and, as I crept, I realized I had that tantalizing Twinkie in my hand at last. You bet I was happy in that moment. Under the bleachers, I looked around like a chimpanzee that just got the last banana off a tree. No one was around. I carefully tore the plastic ribbed top. It opened so gracefully. I could smell it. The yellow cake stuck to my fingers and that white piece of wax paper. I took a moment, smelled it again, and took that first bite. That's when I realized Twinkies taste terrible. What had I done to my reputation for this awful tidbit? I had rebelled against my mother. I could sense my teeth rotting and my mind melting as these guilty thoughts bantered in my conscience. I examined the packaging. Something must be awry. Of course, the expiration date was over a year ago. It was stale, as stale as my own heart.

I ran to find Delilah to protest. She was in the library with her cackle of grackle friends. I went in with a fire in my bones. Her flock dispersed when they saw me coming. It was just me and Delilah. I forgot I was in the library. I took that Twinkie and smashed it right on her awful forehead. She screamed, and the librarian dragged us both to the principal's office. Of course, there was my mother, waiting, and she did not look happy. I was a Twinkie busted bully.

There was a silence on the other end of the phone. "Sarah? You there?"

Sarah returned. "Yes, dear, that is quite the story. Haven't we all a bit of a bully inside us? I have my story to tell as well. May I?"

"Of course." I felt like maybe she did something worse. I hoped to be redeemed by her confession.

Sarah

Sage had his hospitals, and I was chief finance officer of a large phone company. I was second to the boss.

I remember not doing something about a bully. I needed an assistant badly, and internally I knew of a manager, Rachel, who had been with the company for 30 years plus. Rachel was a

GOING THROUGH THE HOOPS

wonderful person. She worked hard, her employees respected and admired her. I asked her if she was interested, and she respectfully declined an executive advancement. I honored that. We did the recruitment and found this pristine younger gal, Jezebel, who had a strong resume'. We hired her.

From day one, she was a tornado of productivity. I noticed Jezebel and Rachel had a somewhat strained relationship. Jez was Rachel's direct supervisor. Rachel stopped coming to meetings and was distant. I called a supervisory meeting with Jez to check in. Jez showed up to my office, literally screaming, "I don't know where you get off calling me in here like you're my mom or something."

I replied, "As your supervisor, I would like to discuss a few things. Is that alright with you?"

She agreed, still huffing and frantically writing things in her planner. She didn't look up much and was as red as a strawberry. This lady was a proud member of a "purple polka-dotted" heritage. Not that it mattered one iota to me. I'm not a judgmental bigot type. I love everyone and respect all for who they are. At least I think I do.

I asked her how Rachel was doing and if she had any concerns. Jezebel looked up and smiled. She told me she felt Rachel was overrated, too well liked by people and ineffective, as well as not that smart. She was thinking of demoting her or putting her on some sort of probation. Something in my tummy told me there was more to the story here. That meeting ended sooner than I'd hoped, but I got what I needed. Immediately after she left, she stomped into the CEO's office and closed the door. Moments later, the CEO came into my office and closed the door. I thought, *What on earth?*

He asked me if I said "As your supervisor" to Jezebel.

I acknowledged that yes, I was her supervisor, and she was emotionally inappropriate.

He said, "I would not have used those words. Your approach is much different from mine." The next day he said he was Jezebel's supervisor going forward; there'd been a change in company policy. He also mentioned under his breath, "She is 'purple polka-dotted', and she mentioned that to me when she came to me. I hope you understand I'm trying to do what is best for our company. We can't have people saying things like we're a prejudiced company. I just wish life was easier. It isn't."

Of course, I did not believe that, and what's wrong with identifying you are someone's supervisor when they are yelling at you? I'd said nothing about her "purple polka-dottiness". She just leveraged it to frighten my boss. Ugh.

I met with Rachel, and she confirmed Jezebel had been oppositional and defeating in their every interaction. Rachel said her work had been criticized to the point she was asking her employees to see it before giving it to Jez, for fear of failure and more verbal railings. She said Jez had called her a "boomer" and "ancient news" behind her back to her employees who came to her concerned. She also said that Jez had especially targeted a young accountant, who just happened to be the same "purple polka-dottiness" and was promising her Rachel's job as soon as the "ole grey mare heads to the farm." I was appalled. Rachel was crying.

I had moments while Rachel was baring her soul and remembered how effective Jez was. She got moved up to the C-suite, given a new office, and scared or blackmailed the CEO as her supervisor and I got chastised. I didn't share that with Rachel, as it was confidential, but everyone kind of knew. Anytime things didn't go Jez's way, she would mutter something about equity and her background. She once said in a speech that companies must not just hire people as a mark on their requirements. She said, "I am not a requirement." It was clear somewhere along the way she had some bad experiences. Well, they weren't with me or my boss, but we were on the receiving end of yet another of her selfish exploits to advance.

Fast forward a couple months. It's the annual employee picnic. I was in my office, and I had a clear view of Jez's new office across the suite from mine. The company had this silly tradition of a hula hoop contest. Rachel was queen of the hoop. She was killing the contest again. You could hear the crowd cheering her on from the courtyard below. The world record is something like 100 hours, but we can't have employees doing that sort of wasteful nonsense, so our company record was 2 hours, and Rachel had the record. That day was special as she only had about 20 minutes to go to beat it once more.

There was an overhead announcement that Rachel was on her way to beating the company record again, to come down to root for Rachel.

Jezebel slammed something on her desk and crashed out of her office like a bull raging after a red flag in a rodeo. I couldn't believe my eyes when I got downstairs. There was Jezebel strapped on with a hula hoop, making snide comments to Rachel, and prodding the crowd to cheer for her instead! How did it come to this? I thought, *Well, I didn't report what I knew then because I, too, was afraid of Jez's newfound friend, the CEO.*

Miriam

"Wow. Isn't it funny, Sarah? I hear stories of this from Ezekiel all the time. How people keep banging into one another."

Sarah sadly commented, "Yes, poor old Sage, my love, couldn't bear it any longer, either. Every good CEO someday must pass that baton—but certainly to earn a good juicy retirement and stock options. Not a darned Twinkie!"

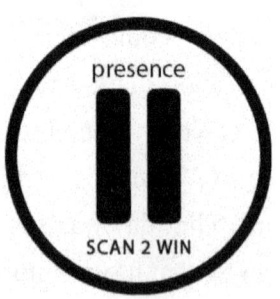

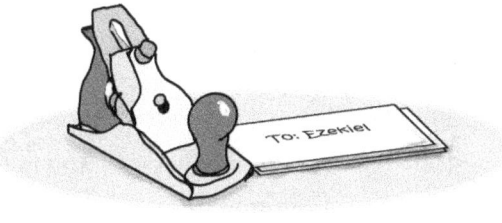

16

Return Recipe to Sender

Ezekiel and Sage

Galatians 6:2 "Carry one another's burdens."

Pearl: "You decide what's truly important."

Ezekiel

I had tucked those 3 envelopes into my briefcase, safe and secure in a zipped pocket. I really didn't want Miriam to see them. So I sat in my wood shop, doodling with a birdhouse, staring at them on my bench. One addressed to Ezekiel. The second addressed to "My Dearest Naomi". The third and final one addressed "Dear God". There was a stain on the one intended for God, and it had a distinct odor of gin still resisting to fade. Why me? I just can't stop thinking, "Why me?"

I dialed up Sage. He answered.

"Sage, I've been given a task to do by a dead man. I really have no recourse but to read the one he addressed to me in simple respect for a man I hardly knew."

Sage quietly grunted. It became my delegated duty. All I knew was Nabal got stuff done, but complained a bit too much. At least that is what people said about him.

"Sage, did you know him?"

Sage answered, "No. I'm afraid he came along after I retired."

"Not everyone liked Nabal," I said. "They all warned me—don't get into deep conversations with Nabal, as he is one that can go on and on. It can get political and dark. He really was a driven kind of guy. His people were sort of afraid of his tirades, or so we've heard. Their collegial advisement and my fatigue from the flight led me to avoid spending time with the man that night. Maybe he was crying out for me to be a friend, and it was a critical point in his life. Did I fail if I didn't know? He was laughing and seemed okay with our rain check. He may have been drinking, and I smelled it. Heck, I went on break to find him. Did he know I was going to do that? Did God? Why me? I feel so stained, Sage. What could I possibly do for him?"

Sage prodded me. "Open the envelope. Let's read it together."

I noticed my hands covered with sawdust and brushed them on my jeans. The powder and puff of dust seemed to linger in the air, just like my anticipatory struggle with the first envelope addressed to me. I held it. I played with its four corners, turned it over, and slid my knife into the crease carefully. Two 3x5 notecards fell out on the bench. Behold. Nabal's manifesto to me. Two 3x5 cards with scribbles on them.

"Sage, there are two cards in the envelope."

Sage asked, "What's on them? You okay?"

I said, "Yeah, I'm fine. The cards say at the top 'FOR ME' and 'FOR THEM.'"

I read the FOR THEM card first. It was a simple message:

1. Get people to think about one another.

2. Get people to pause for one another.

3. Get people to talk to one another.

4. Get people to understand one another.

5. Get people to be curious enough to want to for one another.

I read the FOR ME card. It, too, had a simple message:

1. Forgive me for not thinking.

2. Forgive me for not pausing.

3. Forgive me for not talking.

4. Forgive me for not understanding.

5. Forgive me for not wanting to.

Miriam knocked on the door and pushed it open. She had a picnic tray filled with sandwiches and my favorite chips. Miriam immediately knew I was up to something. She asked, "What's that? Who's on the phone?" I told her it was Sage and asked him if I could call back. He agreed.

I then confessed to Miriam that Nabal had left the envelopes on his bed, and one was addressed to me. She was not thrilled and, contrary to her kindness, blurted, "How dare he? Who are you to him, some work acquaintance? How dare God? Don't they all know what we've been through and are still trying desperately to heal and go on from?"

I thought, *She's been with me a long time and knows my military history. It's her history as well, and our present reality of Abel's addiction. We decided together it was best to leave the Army because of suicides and my role as a commander.*

I said, "Miriam, he had been drinking gin. Lots of it."

She really didn't like that.

She snatched the card, and I let her read. She and I wept together. We seem to share that sentiment being together married all these years. She has a good heart.

She then noted there were two others and warned, "You best not open the one to his wife! Not your place."

I replied, "I'm not God either."

"What's your plan?"

I said I didn't know. We ate our sandwiches in a void that could not be filled. Every now and then, the heater in the garage would rattle out some warm, stale air.

She finally said, "I'm going back to the house now. You should call Sage back. Please don't do anything you might regret. I will pray for us."

I called Sage. "Sage, that was some bad timing. It was my fault. I really should have told Miriam about the envelopes. You know we veterans don't talk about war, and we don't like those crucial conversations about life issues."

Sage said, "Yes, we as humans are not very good at either of those, even if we're not military. So, what's next, Rookie?"

"I don't know. The first thought that popped into my head was to give the one addressed to God to a preacher. I was going to ask Miriam to take a trip with me. Make it a vacation of sorts. Do some deep thinking and talking about our future and what is important to us while we are tourists in unknown lands. Maybe we could swing by Nabal's home and deliver the one to Naomi and leave. What do you think?"

"That's a potential plan," Sage said. "I sense you are considering another life change for yourself and family?"

"Perhaps. I've been doing this work thing for a while now. Don't tell Miriam or Sarah, but my cardiologist is concerned about the level of stress and put me on some new medication. He gave me an antianxiety medication and a safety bottle of nitro."

"Hmmm..."

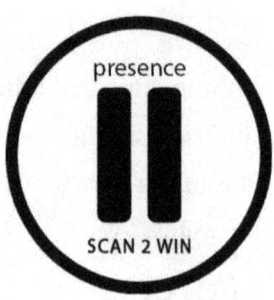

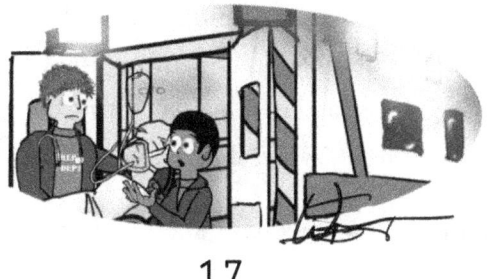

Jimmy...if I may offer a suggestion..."Staying Alive" is more reassuring to the family than "Another One Bites the Dust"...

17

Road Trip and Roadside Stop

Ezekiel and Miriam.

Romans 12:10 "Be devoted to one another."

Pearl: "Life is short, and a gift. Unwrap it like every day is Christmas morning."

Ezekiel

Miriam said to me, "Honey, this was a great idea. So pretty this time of year in the fall. Just look at those leaves and the grand Mississippi River. It's so green and blue. These cliffs are magnificent. Oh, look, a cheese shop, and antiques! Can we?"

"For sure, love. Let's do it."

It was a "blursday", as we had nothing in the planner, and I ditched my work phone. We were alone and together. We decided to explore before getting a snack. I don't recall much else. There was a bit of a hill to get from the parking lot to the shops. I was a little gassed when we got to the top. I thought, *Should I tell Miriam? Nah, it's just indigestion.*

"Oh, look, there's the cheese counter and I see they have Slim Jims!"

Those were the last words I heard Miriam say. How did I wind up in a backwoods hospital bed? What had happened? Was there an angel singing? I could hear my favorite hymn, "How Marvelous." It was Miriam. She was singing it. My eyes started opening wider through the crust, and there was Miriam with a man I'd never met in green surgery scrubs and a priest. *I'm dead. I must be.*

Miriam shouted, "Oh, thank God, Zeke! You're here with us still. This is Father Bill and Dr. Daniel. You had a heart attack, dear. I was so worried."

I had a what?! Not me. No, not possible, I thought. *A heart attack? Oh, my God, my chest hurts. My throat feels like someone pushed a watermelon through it. I'm so dry. Can I have something to drink? What for? A heart attack. We're on vacation. We were looking at cheese. Huh? Am I really in a hospital?*

Miriam said, "The doctor says you'll be okay, but you need to slow down—a lot. You just came out of surgery a few hours ago. You needed a quadruple bypass."

Was I dead or dreaming? Was I still in my office and all of this was not reality? Nope, there stood Father Bill, a priestly kid who looked younger than Abel.

"Here, dear," Miriam said. "I have a hard candy in my purse. Your throat must be so dry from the intubation." That candy was like manna to my spirit. Was I done for? I should just be done.

As Miriam dug in her purse, an envelope fell out on the bed. It was the one addressed, "Dear God". Father Bill saw it and coyly asked, "Is that for me?"

Heck, no better luck than this, I thought. I mumbled through the fading anesthesia and xerostomia bad breath. "Yes, Father, I can explain."

Miriam took over and told him the whole story. He accepted the duty as he proclaimed, "I have a direct channel to the big guy upstairs, being a priest and all." He asked if he should share it with us.

I thought, *Are we reading God's mail, or is he reading us mine?*

Miriam said, "You're a priest. I'm sure if God leads you to share it with us, it's perfectly okay. We were on our way to deliver another note to the author's wife. It's all so very sad."

All I could hear was the incessant beeping of the monitors and my gaze switched rapidly between my lovely Miriam, the priest, and the EKG monitor line. I was intermittently bothered by the hissing of the oxygen canula slipping in and out of my nose. My chest really hurt.

Miriam was watching the rebellious tube and me like a mother eagle, constantly readjusting the plastic hatchling back into my nostril nest. I guess that's all she could control at the time, and it seemed to make her feel useful.

I prayed that the EKG line wouldn't go flat. I felt a tickle in my throat; then it turned into a fire. I coughed. Oh, my God, that was the most pain I ever had. That must be what child birthing is like, or at least it's got to be in the family.

The male nurse came in, tearing plastic off a red heart-shaped pillow and gave it to me to clutch. I grabbed that thing with a vengeance.

He said, "This little guy will be your best friend for a while now, Zeke. No more crazed board room meetings for you for a while, either—maybe never. You need to listen to what we say. You're not the CEO in here, buddy. Hear me? Oh, by the way, your cortisol levels were ridiculous. Doc has a lot to tell you about what you need to change."

I knew he was being funny, and I thanked him for the pillow, but what was to be next for me? For Miriam? For Abel? What the heck is cortisol?

Father Bill took out a pen from his pocket and slipped it through the crease of the envelope, and sure enough, another 3x5 card emerged.

ROAD TRIP AND ROADSIDE STOP

Father Bill quietly read it to himself, then recited it aloud:

"FOR MANKIND

1. Thank you for forgiving us.

2. Thank you for feeding us.

3. Thank you for healing us.

4. Thank you for saving us.

5. Why didn't you save me from doing this?"

After a long silence, with only the hospital sounds buzzing, beeping, and hissing, Father Bill said, "This last envelope should be delivered soon, and you folks won't be leaving this hospital for at least a week. May I offer to deliver Naomi's?" Miriam handed Father Bill the last envelope.

So, there we were, alone. Miriam and me, my cortisol cocktail, and cardiac cushion. She lost it. Sobbing, chastising, thanking, silently screaming, and then nothing. My Miriam never swore a day in her life. This was worse than our worst marital tiff. She was always the picture of poise and kindness. Her voice could cut through ice fog with words that were straight from her core. I listened this time. I listened well. I understood. I was curious to learn more from her.

She said, "Ezekiel, I don't want to read a letter from you. Do you understand?"

Tears filled my eyes. My heart felt new and ready. My legs trembled, although I was lying in a bed. I gently held her hand and said, "I do."

She pulled Ryder's coin from her purse and placed it in our hands, and we held it and each other. We put on the full armor of God.

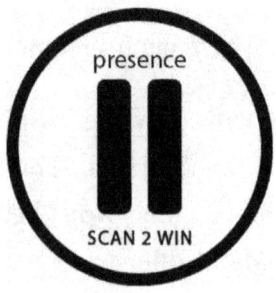

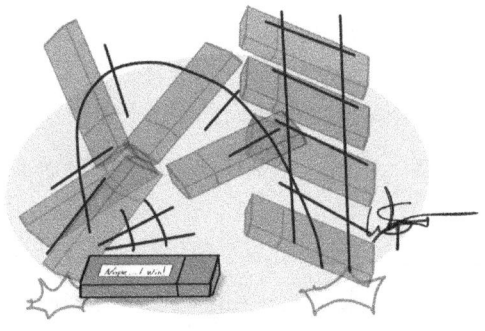

18

The Rest of the Story

Ezekiel and Sage

Ephesians 4:2 "Be humble toward one another in love."

Pearl: "Take time to build, and less time to tear it down."

Ezekiel

Miriam slipped outside my hospital room door to make a couple phone calls. I could overhear her because she always puts her cell on speaker. One was to Abel, which did not end well.

She started, "Hello, son. Your father is okay, but he had a massive heart attack. We're going to go to an old friend's home to recover. It's not far from you."

It was his birthday, and he was drinking heavily. He muttered and slurred out, "Thank you for blaming me for this too on my birthday. You two are priceless." For some reason, he has taken the weight of the world upon his shoulders and can't escape these delusions of doom. He moved out of our house, and we know he's struggling. Nothing we can do but pray and try to stay in touch. Miriam said goodbye and we love you, then hung up.

She then called Sarah and told her about my heart attack. Sage was in the background saying, "Tell them to come here for some peaceful rest." Miriam didn't even argue, but graciously thanked Sarah and came back to tell me what I already knew.

I asked Miriam for a paper and a pen. She handed it to me, and I scribed out my letter of resignation/retirement. Her eyes welled up, but we both knew it was time. The doctor said I could be out of this hospital prison the next day; sooner than expected. So, we planned to travel the short trip to Sage's. I felt a wave of resurrection and redemption flowing over me. I had a second chance at life—not work. No more work. Now life. Just life, and life more abundantly. Never to be the same again. Nabal's manifesto. Was that really for me to do something with?

We awoke early and, unlike most rural hospitals, we were discharged and on our way before 8 am. I desperately wanted a fast-food breakfast sandwich, but there was no suggesting that.

Miriam already had a full-on fruit basket for breakfast and black coffee. Thank God for the coffee!

The trip went by quickly, and soon we were on the back county road turning by an old, crooked mailbox into the two-track driveway. The trees sheltered the path, and the sun peeked through like golden lasers through the budding leaves overhead. It was serene. "Oh, look, Zeke, a doe, and her fawn! How precious."

I responded, "Yes, it is a sign of new life and spring." Miriam smiled and put her hand on my knee. We made the turn into the long drive. There was a humble Cape Cod home perched upon a hill with a beautiful, expansive front yard of lush green.

Sage was seated like royalty upon his John Deere tractor and waving as if he was at a Macy's Thanksgiving parade. He jumped off, and Sarah came running to our car simultaneously to greet us. We pretty much all cried together. They were out of breath and Sage was coughing almost as bad as I was. It was emotional. I felt safe and at peace, and I sensed all their gratitude that I was still here with them. That felt good.

We got situated on the back deck, and Sarah and Miriam were in the kitchen scurrying about, laughing. It sounded like it was about the two ole codgers on the deck watching birds. Sage and I had perched ourselves in the cedar Adirondack chairs. We weren't going anywhere anytime soon. We marveled at the woodsy haven they called their summer cottage.

It was 78 degrees and a perfect spring morning. There were at least 50 birdhouses of all shapes and sizes. I lost count at 30 birds of differing species. They were all singing, tweeting, chirping, and screeching. A hummingbird was suspended gracefully right in front of us for a moment, then it darted at the speed of light off to the next flower.

I asked Sage, "Did you build all of those?"

Sage responded, "Yep, it was my self-therapy when I left RHS. Thankfully, I didn't have a heart attack like you, you old fool. I just ran out of gas and patience. While I was working and had a challenge, I would go to the shop and write down my thoughts and plans on the inside of a birdhouse. All of those are filled with my avian wallpaper leadership exploits. Some of my best stuff and craziest plans are in those houses. Some of my deepest thoughts, too. It was my way of winning each day."

I had no idea Sage had left abruptly like his mentee, Jazz, and now me.

"Yes, Sarah couldn't support my working that hard anymore. She retired before me and was happy. I had encountered Satan himself, as my boss, and just could not go on."

"Do you mind sharing what happened?"

Sage began telling a tale of tales, as he always did.

Sage

It was at the pinnacle of my career with RHS. I really had arrived, and things were on autopilot for my hospitals. See, I worked my way up to the corporate level as one of the district CEOs. I proudly led seven RHS systems. They were great people and communities. Patients were our priority and that kept me going. Surprisingly, the board decided to fire our long time CEO and replaced her with her assistant, Ananias.

This guy was top dog now. He knew it and turned out to be an immediate ass. He really was a piece of work—quite the deceiver. No one knew why the board and our top CEO had a falling out. They said it was a difference of vision. News spread through the ranks that Ananias had something to do with exposing the boss for some financial dealings and conflicts. No one wanted to believe it, but they fired her. They had a big party for her going away in Philadelphia, and made it look like it was a voluntary bittersweet departure, but she told some of us closest to her she was fired with no other options and to watch out for Ananias. That's all she said.

From day one with him as my boss, I knew bad was the only outcome. I tried desperately every day to take on a new perspective by burying the lies that kept rising in me. Sure enough, a couple weeks into his reign, nine other CEOs walked or were convinced somehow. Three of them were my direct reports. I was facing a deluge of search committee setups and at least a year of unrest in my hospitals. Okay, RHS wasn't the powerhouse it is now; yet this was a challenge I didn't need.

Anyway, for some reason, he created a renewed "probation" period for everyone in leadership. He and HR had colluded and were now vetting executives his way, and suddenly all of us were "probates". I had over 30 years in and I'm on probation with a solid record?

He started meeting with us all online. Skype just came on the scene, and he loved looking at himself. You could tell because his eyes were never on the straightforward and shifting. You could also see who was in his gang of unfriendliest, too. They would all be looking down at their phones and laughing or smiling when one of us was explaining Ananias's deluded impressions of what he expected from our productivity. Sometimes they messed up and put disparaging remarks in the chat window for all to see. Nothing was ever done about it. One time someone put "That's profiling" when one of my colleagues talked about an active shooter drill and how they have some increased gang activity around their campus. It was ruthless and out of context. He forced us to listen to his berating of our staff and productivity. He never once mentioned the word "patient". Ananias was all about himself and the bottom line—more money. I kept my internal message to not become a slave to him or my thoughts.

I despised that about him, and it probably came through over the computer screen. One day, about six months in, he called a private meeting with me at his corporate office. I flew into Philadelphia and, well, it did not turn out to be the city of brotherly love for me. He downgraded my position, and I was now just a clinic practice manager. Ananias just re-wrote it and said I was out of the CEO business. He said I could compete for it if I wanted to. He also said I would have to relocate to Philadelphia. Then he added, "But there are others who will give you a run for your money, so don't have your hopes high."

For six months, he just kept sending me email after email of the little things he saw me doing he didn't agree with and demanded I change and provide him with evidence. He also pressured me to rush the searches and fill the walk-away CEO positions. He blamed me and my poor leadership attention to what was important: profits.

When I returned from Philly, I was greeted that morning by his self-appointed henchwoman who was now my "personal professional assistant". Her name was Rahab. Rahab was a looker. She handed me a memorandum from the board that appointed her as part of my probationary period to help observe and assist with systems redesign. She was a Black Belt LEAN Six Sigma and had a PhD in organizational development on paper. In theory, I was grateful for the help she might bring with that pedigree of hers. In practice, she was much less effective. She followed me everywhere, with clipboard in hand, diligently jotting things as she called it. I heard her every morning reviewing the list with Ananias and giggling. They were indeed flirtatious. It got so bad that Ananias had Rahab meet with him weekly, and she then briefed me on his expectations. I was out of his loop. I knew I had to maintain my focus daily to stay sane. If there was one word that defines me at my best, it is "focused".

She interviewed my entire staff, and afterward, people were quite distant from me. People started talking like there was something going on between us. Absolutely not!

Rookie, let me tell you how Sarah and I met. I was strong in everything except for girls. I would sweat profusely just seeing someone I was attracted to. Sarah was beyond attraction. She was spectacular. It was a rainy day, and she was running into a restaurant. She slipped, and her books went everywhere. I ran to her rescue, scooped her up gently, and carried her into the restaurant. I then went outside and got her books. That was a bold moment for me, but then my inner bully scared me, and I only said, "I'm glad you're okay. Can I have your phone number?" Then I ran off. I did get her number. So, I called her a few days later and asked her, "How is the weather?" At our wedding, our song and my daily wake-up song is "Happy Together" by the Turtles. There's a lyric that mentions "picking up a dime to call and ask about the weather"! That's exactly what I did, and here we are happy together decades later.

Anyway, it was the other way around. My boss and Rahab, who previously worked in HR, were now his on-site spies. They were the ones carrying on. How did I know this? Well, my revised position downgrade and notification were signed by the HR classification supervisor—you guessed it, Rahab! *How much more blatant can it get?* I thought. She didn't let me out of her sight. One time she was waiting for me outside the executive washroom, tapping her foot and looking at her fancy Rolex. I had had it. Being with RHS for so many good years, I called a buddy of mine who just happened to have retired recently from the board. He said he would mention the indiscretions to the chair of the board who was an honest lady and suggest an investigation.

It worked... well, sort of. The investigation began. Ananias was placed on an administrative sabbatical, still getting paid. Rahab was still filling him in on happenings. I asked her once if she was in contact with him and she got HR to put a restraining order on me, as she felt retaliated against.

When it concluded, all the bones of their skeleton came crawling out of the closet. Rahab and Ananias's affair, the abuse of power, and the forced or coerced departures of the other CEOs. I found out they all testified. It appeared things were going to be better.

No one knows why, but the board put that devil back in the seat. I became hopeless and suicidal. Sarah and I were in counseling. It was dark, my friend, very dark. My position was still downgraded, and I was still in the interview process to compete for my downgraded job. No one would talk to me because they feared the wrath of Ananias. I was alone. One panelist on the search team was Rahab's uncle. You guessed it; I didn't even get an interview.

Our daughter taught me how to make a video and encouraged me to do one for my profile on a headhunter website in the face of the inevitable loss of my job. So, I was in the process of making that video when Ananias came into my office. It was tense. I turned off my monitor so he wouldn't see what I was doing. He shut the door. He didn't sit down. I remember his patronizing look. It was disgusting and prideful, as though no one could touch him. He was full of himself.

He said to me, "I know you're dying, old man. You're dying in this job, and you are killing the organization with all these 'breaks' to take shots. What's up with that? How are you making up that time lost? I haven't seen any requests or records of this abuse of sick leave. We will have to talk more about this. Bottom line here, geezer, is there's only room for one CEO around here. Sage, you probably should consider that carefully the next time you go to mommy and daddy. I'm going to be successful with or without you. Rahab and I are getting married, so you can stop the gossiping, old man, and get back to work. I win. I will always win. Get that in your head." He left.

I sat staring, fuming, and ready to pounce at the injustice. Just then, I looked up at my computer and it was recording! I closed my door and replayed the recording, and it was all there. I called my daughter, and she told me how to save it on a flash drive. His surreptitious abuse was not so secret now. Of course, this confession of sorts couldn't be used in court, but I did send the recording to the board for their further consideration of his harassment and intentions. I specifically inquired about my medical records and who had accessed them, because how could Ananias know about my diabetes and cancer treatments?

Something came over me Rookie, like a transformation. I knew I had him by the short ones. I made another copy on a flash drive and took out a Sharpie and wrote, "Nope, I win" on the red plastic cover. I pushed my chair back and headed down the hall to the conference room where Ananias had set up his temporary office. He was at the table with his feet up on one of the leather chairs. It was my chair at the head of the table. He was polishing his shoes, which were black. Our chairs were light tan leather. There were traces of polish on my chair.

I inquired, "Sir, do you have a quick moment? I would like to give you our latest metrics on antimicrobial stewardship and length of stay improvements. We've done quite well. I have it here on a flash drive for your convenience."

He popped up and said, "You know how to make a flash drive? I suppose you even have a flip phone." I conceded I needed to learn more about technology, but yes, I did do this. He then pulled out his laptop and plugged in the flash without even looking at it. Once he hit the open button, the recording played. He was enraged. He said, "You'll never be able to use any of this! You broke the law recording me! Oh, I got you now, buddy." Then he threw the flash drive at my face.

I caught it, and I thought, *Bless my daughter*. She told me that the recording was a "mike drop moment". So, yep, indeed, I did just that. I held that flash up in the air above his head, dropped that flash drive on his laptop, and told him to read the cover.

He read it out loud. "Nope, I win." I told him the board already had a copy of the drive.

In good ole fashioned Paul Harvey style, I said, "Get this in your head Ananias... I win...and that...Ananias, is the rest of the story."

I left.

Like I suspected, they found one of Rahab's friends, who was a nurse that was never involved in my care, had accessed oncology and endocrinology reports. They fired Ananias and Rahab on the same day. Police walked them out together. It was glorious and terribly sad all at once. You would think that was my relief. No, it was my wake-up call to go make birdhouses. I realized I was not the best version of me that was possible. So, I did—I up and left.

Ezekiel

I said, "Sage, that was some saga you went through. I had no idea you were ill. Are you still?"

"Yes, I'm fighting it. See the port? Sarah takes me for treatments weekly. It's a matter of time."

"I'm so sorry."

Sage said, "I smoked a bit too much, I guess. Started in my lungs. Now it's pretty much everywhere. The treatments are keeping it at bay, and they give me a lot of good meds for the pain."

"Sage, what do you make of this manifesto of Nabal's?"

Sage stalled a bit and said, "I think we will have to do something about it. It's got to be a better culture, or we're all doomed. I think Nabal probably knew he wasn't his best self, either."

I agreed. But what?

Miriam and Sarah appeared and handed Sage the hot dogs and burgers to put on the grill. He promptly became the back yard male version of Julia Child, screeching out with a terrible English accent while he put on his "Best grandpa ever" apron, with spatula and tongs in hand. Tons of character and goodness in this man. I adored him and it hurt, thinking he might be gone someday soon. The smell of the burgers and dogs was relaxing, and once the wives sat down, they began small talk.

Sarah started, "We are all so fortunate to be here, happy together today. I'm very thankful we met at Tahoe. Seems our paths are very similar."

Miriam piped in, "Yes, we are birds of a feather, the four of us. We're so grateful for your invitation. It is time we just relax and take a deep breath. So many birds!"

Sage entered from his sentry position at the grill. "I don't see this as an accident. We need to celebrate Rookie's retirement! I'm going to call a few people and invite them. Are you both okay with a little soiree? I didn't get a party myself. It could be for both of us."

At first, I was reluctant, but could see right through Sage's intention. He was so strategic. I said, "Yeah, that sounds great to see people who are not busy at a conference or meeting. Just enjoying one another."

Sage handed me the barbeque tools and rushed off into his den to make calls. He has a bellowing voice at times, and the first thing we heard through the patio door was, "Hey Esther, how are you doing these days?" We could hear Esther's enthusiasm, and I kept watch on the burgers and dogs. Sarah and Miriam started working on ideas for snacks and guessing how many might be coming to the soiree.

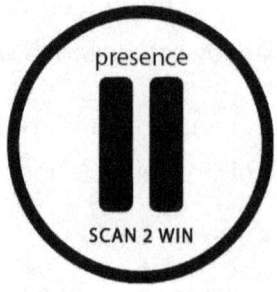

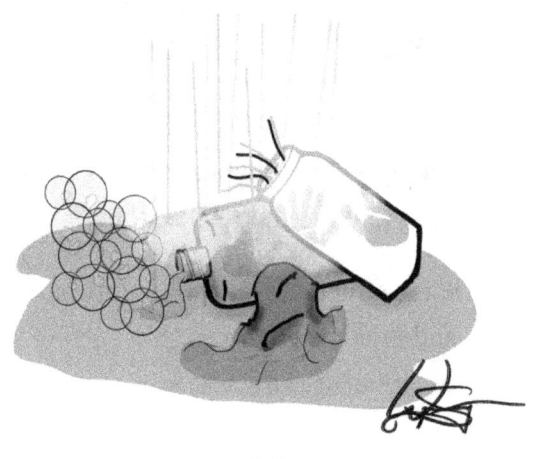

19

Mine!

Rahab and Yovanna

Philippians 2:4: "Let not every man look upon his own things, but also on the things of others."

Pearl: "What's mine is yours."

Rahab

The rain was pounding on the metal roof of the Airstream. It seemed to take all my energy to count the individual pings and to stir their lunch. It wasn't much, but it was a shelter of sorts I had landed in. I held the pot in one hand and wiped my brow with the other. It was hot and humid, due to the rain and the AC... Oh yeah, there is no AC. I live in a tuna can now. I guess I'm thankful for it. Back in the day, this Airstream was high class.

Certainly, this silver bullet is not the executive lavish life I once had in the hills of Nashville, Tennessee. I wish I had a silver bullet now to kill the vampire that sucked the life out of me. Me.

I remember when it rained there; it was so beautiful. Ananias and I would sit and look out the huge glass picture windows at the trees and grass growing. Life was good then. I had arrived. My family. My business. My friends. My money——oh, the money! My service to those who needed me. Social work and mental health were my life and dream. People followed me.

I worked at RHS as a youngster. I learned my way under a psychologist. I was a proud clinical assistant. I was self-made. I didn't have the pedigree of the other clinical staff, but I had the business ideas and the guts to open the venture.

The day I bought a failing business, my last thought would have been that I would have something to do with it failing a second time. My family was on board. They invested hard-earned savings to support and join me. It became our reality——our family dream. It was a place of work, but a home for family and friends to mingle and make some dough. Not Play-Doh.

I had it all. Why could I not see that then? I wanted it all, and it was mine at the time.

Oh, those boys! Why do they fight so much? "Jesus, please help me today", I prayed. I hadn't prayed in quite some time, but I knew I could use a hand. The intensity of the two boys screaming, "Mine, mine, mine!" was like a tornado siren in my ears. I had to see what was going on. I didn't really want to know.

I walked down the narrow mobile home hallway, carrying the pot of mac and cheese to their bedroom. Ugh! There was another leak in the roof!

My 2-year-old twin boys, Perez and Zerah, were on the floor in the middle of the room mixing baby powder, Mr. Bubble, and Play-Doh on the white carpeting. Red Play Doh.

The constant flood of water pouring out of the leak had increased and had become a steady stream. There were chunks of ceiling tile on their heads and on the floor. It was swelling like a strained ankle. The boys squealed while shoving each other under the stream and into the mess they created on the floor. Rolling in it, scrambling for more. It was all over them; in their hair, on their clothes and embedded in the carpet. They both wanted to be in the mess, so they kept screaming, "Mine". I just cried, thinking, *Where's mine?*

I couldn't believe it had come down to this. I'd lost everything. I didn't have a life. I had given it away. I was blind and too proud and stingy.

I was Rahab, or at least I thought I was. I was a successful businesswoman owner. I was married. I was happy. I had a lot of friends. I was in control. I had a lot of money and stuff. We had a life, and it was awesome.

Now I live in a trailer, barely scraping mac and cheese off the bottom of the pot to make ends meet for me and my boys. What happened?

The sounds of the twins faded as I did too. I leaned against the wood-paneled hallway wall, cascading back to a rainy night four years ago. My mental movie began:

It all started in Yovanna's Lexus. I was impressed with her. She was a new woman to the company, but she was smart, held big degrees and broad experience. She intimidated me some internally, but I wanted to be like her.

Her hubby, Joel, already worked for us, and he was good. He had bounced back after surviving a bout with cancer. He transformed our social media presence and marketing. Joel got our name on the streets and with top psychologists and psychiatrists in the region. He was talented. We all knew it and trusted and supported him through the disease. He told our team about Yovanna, his wife, and that we could have her join as our CFO/COO. It was a no-brainer for me—I hired her. Yovanna was seeking a new opportunity, and she longed for a different pace than the large corporate finance world. We were a good fit.

We had just finished a business presentation at a major marketing conference where she presented for our company. I never asked her to vet the talk with me, because I had assumed she was so well put together it would be fine. I didn't like what or how she did it. I gave her our power point. I do it the same way every time——my way.

On the ride home, I began the conversation, telling her all the things I would have done differently. She seemed guarded. I didn't pay attention to the clues of how my tone was being received. I don't know, anyway, I was talking and talking, maybe too much. My excitement may have gotten the best of me. I expected different. I expected her to present just like I would have. Why would she have changed it? Who did she think she was? The company was mine. Yovanna joined my team as chief operating officer (COO), and she rapidly drove our finances to the next level. She may not have been a good front person. She was a true go-getter. A forgetful one, but highly capable. But this presentation concerned me.

We got several more referrals than usual out of her presentation. More than I ever got. I became jealous. I could feel the burning in my stomach; it was spiteful. I didn't like how she achieved and was resentful her approach worked. It was the first time in her first year, and I had fears and doubts that Yovanna was out to get my company and my position. I had to get control and keep control. Ananias was aloof to it all. He never really did anything, but I had to add him to get the loan. He loved marching around in his pin-striped suits, acting like a big shot.

To make matters worse, my college roomie, Hedda, oversaw the administrative support teams and scheduling of patients. She had told me many times of her concern that billing and scheduling weren't on track with one another. I ignored that. I only gave her the easy jobs I knew she could handle, but she was my alum. It was nice having her nearby. We would often sneak off to one of the clinics and have extended lunches. I sure enjoyed Hedda's company, and she was always a wealth of information about staff. She seemed to know a bit more than I liked her to about Ananias, as well. Hedda really didn't understand what the schedulers do, but I lent a hand when I saw things getting rough.

The company grew so much and very quickly. We had 16 employees, and in one year of Yovanna's influence, we arrived at 200 and were still expanding. Forty of those were admin and were supervised by Hedda. I knew Hedda was overwhelmed, but I couldn't fire her. She had just divorced and had been down on her luck for a few years. Hedda liked to spend her money. She was always nicely dressed. She had taste in fashion. We loved shopping together. She out bought me in every boutique.

When things got remarkably lucrative, I wanted more of my pie. I asked Yovanna to increase my salary, yet not appear out of range with others. I felt I could trust her and was doing her a favor, too. I told her to pay my hubby, Ananias, a salary and to give herself a 5% raise. That padded our overall home incomes. Ananias was a loser from the start. I knew he'd fail us somehow, someday. He did. Hedda was my friend. Ananias is wearing a different striped suit nowadays!

The slide began when Hedda and I were at lunch one day. She blamed Yovanna for some serious income loss due to poor billing oversight. She did not like her. I was intimidated by Yovanna and must have been locked in fear of her abilities and presence. At any rate, I started conversations with Yovanna, and that's how it went down. I had to have the upper hand with her. Yovanna and her hubby just up and left one day. Six months after they left, I filed for bankruptcy, and here I am in the silver bullet. I wonder what the tipping point was. If only I could have been a fly on the wall in Yovanna's head.

"Okay, boys. Mommy is back." The water slowed, and I decided to just sit down with them on the floor. We all ate mac n cheese out of the pot. The boys thought that was fun. I thought, *They're mine alright. They're mine.*

Yovanna

(Six months ago... Yovanna leaving Rahab's office.)

I'm glad this wall is here for me to lean on. I can barely stand. What just happened? She really laid into me this time. Those were threats. I've never felt so small and so big at the same time. How did I let her have this power over me? Did she steal it from me?

Rahab is an absolute fool. She's made me so confused. I don't know where I fit in this company anymore. My team is equally confused. My budget staff members are so distant, and I don't know why. They very rarely get reports to me. They say that Rahab assigned those reviews to Ananias. I thought that was part of my job. She just keeps changing things. It's madness. What am I doing wrong? Why don't I fit? What could I do better? Why do I fail so much in her eyes?

Hedda is a terrible leader, and she doesn't get the negative supervisory attention I get. She gets coddling. What if she wants to fire me? I have no recourse. I really must tell Joel. We need a plan. I'll just get started reviewing these accounts. Yovanna, put on your big girl pants now and carefully look at her money. My sanity is mine.

I said to him, "Joel, honey, we've got to talk. Today Rahab called me into her office and rained a bomb down on me. She put me on a performance improvement plan (PIP). I'm destroyed. I've never been questioned by any boss before. I think you know Hedda set this up. You've been working with them. What do you think? Do you see it as possible? I told Rahab I had concerns about Hedda, and that our clinicians were not being fully utilized. We've got clients on waiting lists and open appointment availability. What gives?"

Joel responded, "I just do the marketing. I am good at it, and there are a lot of new referral sources and more coming. I've wondered about staffing ratios to incoming patients. You seem upset and frustrated. Sit down here and tell me more."

I continued, "I just don't know. It's been a year of hell. She keeps needling me. She berates, belittles, excludes me from meetings... She'll talk to you, and now she's even stopped speaking to you. Now a PIP! I don't deserve this. All I am doing is my job. We're going to sink financially soon. We can't meet payroll, and Rahab knows it. She blamed me. She said I have not done well with the billing oversight. I'm worried. Maybe I should start looking for another job. I've reviewed all the past monthly reports and we're just not working up to capacity. There are some minor coding errors, but those don't add up to being in the red like we are—millions. In my estimation, we've got maybe four months of surplus to survive. She'll have to sell, or worse."

Joel said, "Hmm. I had no idea. This is not good. We still need the healthcare coverage. I'm still on chemo treatments. Ya know, last week she stopped by my office and mentioned that all the leadership team should be thinking of a Plan B, as we are looking at some organizational changes, she called it. She was acting weird; like excited, but not. I chalked it up to her usual wishy-washy personality. Didn't think much of it. She left, saying she was thankful I'm getting better."

"There's more to this," I said. "I'm certain. She said that Hedda was concerned that my billing department and her scheduling departments were not working well together. I informed her we have a weekly huddle and that I was the lead. She said she was going to be the lead going forward, and that I am reduced to her special assignments, starting with checking every single ledger item in accounts payable and receivable. She said she lost confidence in my ability, and that was the reason for the PIP.

"She asked me if I had counseled or assisted any of Hedda's employees. I said that they often will approach me or my supervisors about open slots in the schedule. We do guide them when possible. She turned purple, Joel. Next, she asked me why I added a 5% raise to my salary. Can you believe that? I did not tell her we decided against it. Joel, I lied to her to see what she would say next. I don't trust her. Sure enough, she said she was kidding, and to immediately reimburse the company, as I clearly misunderstood her. We knew that was one of her spontaneous moments. Thank God we didn't take the raise. I did add her hubby's, however, per her direction. I sent her an email, too, verifying the promotion. She said, 'You know that is embezzlement to some eyes. Fix it.' She dismissed me from her office, muttering under her breath, 'This company is still mine.'"

Joel said, "Wow, that is worse than I'd imagined. Sounds like she fears you. I'm thinking about a change too. I'd like to start my own consulting business. Maybe now is the time? Let's pursue our dreams. Hopefully, we can secure healthcare insurance soon. It will take some time to get consulting off the ground."

I said, "I've already sent out resumes! I texted my old boss, too. What I'm about to share with you is astonishing, but it's a fact. In reviewing all my homework for Rahab, I've discovered that Ananias has been working with Hedda, and they are placing interdepartmental fake purchase orders in the millions of dollars, a little at a time. In fact, I'm embarrassed I hadn't seen this earlier, or any of my team, for that matter. He is getting rich on the side, or they are, while Rahab parades around like royalty, bullying some of us. I'd imagine Hedda is too. The company would be well in the black with that money. We still are not productive. We should be hugely successful."

Joel said, "You know she and Hedda went to the same college or something. What are you going to do about this?"

"I don't know," I said. "I think we should just leave this ship before it takes a real dive. There's a hole in it, and a flood of failure is pouring through it. It's all about to come down on her head and she's too blind to see it. We have an audit next week. They will find this. Well, I will have to show this to them, or I'm going to be held culpable. She's already trying to blame me. It's her own family and friends who are deceiving her. The audit will uncover that, too. She sure acted like a 2-year-old——mine, mine, mine... I want to leave right after the audit is completed. I tried to help. I tried to show her. She hated me or something. I feel sorry for her. I don't feel sorry about how she has treated me. Joel, what do you think?"

Joel said, "The decision is ours. Yours and mine."

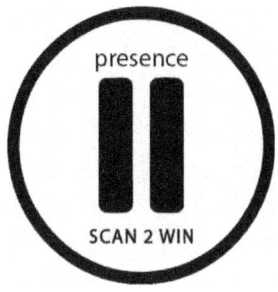

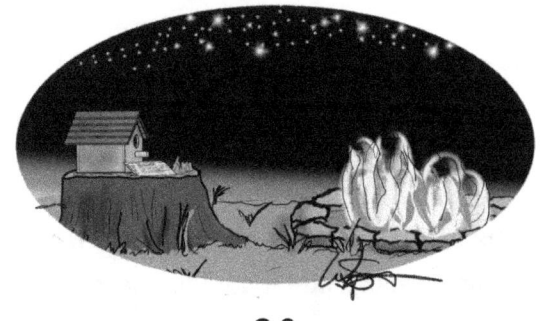

20

Birdhouse Bullies

Sage and Sarah

Nehemiah 6:2: "But they thought to do me mischief."

Pearl: "If you never go where you've never been, you will end up where you are."

Sage

"Sarah, I've called everyone, and the list is about 40 total overall. The first group is all our CEO friends. You remember my mentor, Jonah? He was a white coat and bowtie guy. He always had the most colorful ones. That guy's still kicking at 92, and he said he's coming! He still has a private practice. Won't that be a hoot for all the gang to meet him?"

Sarah said, "Sage, you've outdone yourself. Now rest."

"I think I will do that. I'm going to go out to the shop and doodle a bit. Call me when Ezekiel and Miriam are awake. We can have a nice brunch together. The guests will start pouring in after one o'clock."

I sat in my neglected shop, pondering. I knew I had to take the lead in brainstorming, and it couldn't be Zeke. He was still recovering. *Good thing Miriam gave me those two 3x5 cards. That will be a good place to start. What a sad story. I'm sure everyone will have something to say about Nabal and what happened. What is this about? What about this is important to me? To all of us? Is it about all of us or all of them? For me, for them, for God? What did Nabal mean by all of this and that?*

The shop was a dustbin, so I started cleaning up a bit. There's never a moment I come out here I don't find something to do. Never ending. *Stay focused, Sage. Well, look at that, I've been wondering where that house went*, I thought. It had been under these rolls of paper all these years. It's the first one I started and never finished. What an ugly mess it is! Hardly my best work.

Under the dust were faded writings. I remembered this was the darkest of days for me when I attempted the first house build. I carefully wiped all the dust off and there revealed my thoughts in green Sharpie: "Build with and upon one another. Don't destroy one another." On the inside of the roof, I see another nugget: "People aren't broken, and I don't have to fix them." I must have been drinking truth serum to come up with that one. There was something else on the floor of this old house: "The gifts and calling of God are without repentance." I remember that one well. I held onto the without repentance part.

I knew I was good for RHS, and it was good for me. I was so depressed, losing that old friend. I spent many days and nights catering to it and making sure our patients got safe and quality healthcare—they were my family, too. I loved my mission and without it, I would have been lost if it wasn't for Sarah.

Was there something there we might all be missing? Was it right before my eyes? "The gifts and calling." I wondered if I'd ever used my gifts against someone. *They sure used theirs against me. Well, sure I did. I was not very kind to Ananias in return. Hell, he deserved what he got. Didn't he? Maybe that is the secret sauce here. Maybe we all deserve what we get? We all have a choice to bully or be bullied? Do we all have to dish it out and then take it? Why do we dish it out at all? Hey, that's not a bad place to start this off with the 3x5 cards and some group talk. Do we start each day losing and striving to win or setting our mindset to win for the right reasons?*

I decided to cut out ten birdhouses so we could sit around the fire, having s'mores and writing our thoughts about the subject, combining our efforts. Everyone would get to take their house home with them; a memento and reminder of what we came up with. I was confident this group of brilliant humans would discover something to help make the world a better place.

Sarah yelled, "Sage! Brunch! Come and get it."

I loaded up the John Deere with all the wood, paints, brushes, sandpaper, and tools and headed up to the house. We sat in the sunroom together having our coffee and quiche. Nervously, I shared my bird-brained birdhouse idea. The ladies loved it. Rookie was not all in.

He said, "Do you really think that these professionals will do this? Write their thoughts on a piece of wood?" Zeke was a verbal processor. Zeke said, "Hey, wait a minute. I have something in my briefcase my EA gave me to investigate using with our team. Oh, here it is! It's a thing from the Dream Leader Institute (DLI). It's called 'Win the Day'. Sage, I think we should start the group off with this. It covers mission, gratitude, focus, self-improvement, and affirmation. I was drawn to this, but, well, we all know what happened to me." I nodded. "That's what we all want, is to know our purpose and grow into the greatest version of ourselves as leaders and people."

"I don't know, but learning is something that happens best when it is novel. I can't think of anything more novel, and not like some boring conference, than writing on a bunch of sticky notes and plastering the walls in our home. Can you? Aren't we all more creative when we're creating something?"

Miriam piped up and said, "I love it. Birdhouses for Bullies!"

"Zeke, what do you think?" I asked. "Good plan? Win the day. Rid the bullies?"

Zeke replied, "I believe you're on to something that will help us all be great."

BIRDHOUSE BULLIES

We finished brunch. As we were cleaning up, the first guests arrived. Esther rolled up in her 1972 Volkswagen van with flower power. She planned on tenting. Luke rumbled in on his Harley Davidson. He said he was sleeping under the stars in a mummy bag. A pristine black Model A Ford appeared from the dust of Luke's bike. Proudly driving it, and blasting his aooooogah horn was Jonah, still the life of the party at 92! The horn was blasting, and he had his head out the window, yelling, "Aoooogah" at everybody!

There wasn't a single colored hair on his head. He still had a long, unruly mop of hair. It was as metallic as a Susan B. Anthony silver dollar. He was equally old as her. *He kind of resembles Einstein*, I thought. His bow tie was the best I'd ever seen. It was custom-made. It was black and white and had little gravestones with "RIR" written on them. I asked him about the RIR, and he said: "WWWW-Why that is for 'RRRRRest in RRRRRetirement'!" I knew we were in for a pun extravaganza.

See, Jonah had stuttered from birth. He used a compensatory strategy of stuttering on purpose and puns to distract and push through some moments in his speech. Jonah is the most intelligent man I've ever met. He introduced me to birding. He was my professor and a friend.

Ruth came in her convertible mini with her two navigator huge Afghan hounds in the passenger seat, named Raja and Bubba. The gang was all here! Well, minus one.

I felt bad about what I did to Ananias. Behold, I got a call just last week from him asking if I would be willing to give a reference for him. We had a good talk. I invited him to join us a day early with the team. After all, who would know bullies better than the best one I ever met? He offered an olive branch; but he needed something. I was still a bit wary of his wares, but I took it for what it was worth to do the right thing, and I forgave him. He forgave me as well. I hoped he would come.

I wanted Rookie to have a splendid retirement, and to have a strong group of minds to work out this manifesto. There would be no talk of cancer. Just joy and focus. This group is always so good at focus.

The fire was blazing, and everyone was having a great time together. We finished an amazing tournament of bags, and the pulled pork went over fantastic. Time for s'mores.

I said, "Friends, I've asked you here a day early so we can put our heads together on something important. I want us to make birdhouses together!" You could hear a pin drop. Maybe Ezekiel was right, and we should have started with his worksheets.

Then Ruth said, "What a splendidly fun thing. Why are we doing this?"

"Well," I said. "We all have heard about Nabal and his ending his life. He left us something. Not us, but Ezekiel. He found Nabal in his room, and he was given these cards. It's a manifesto of sorts, we think. We all know the bullying in our lives and organization. Nabal's life and work should not be in vain. He gave us some things to think about and I think we darn well should do something about it. What do you say? Are you in for a good ole fashioned brainstorming s'more session?"

Jonah interjected, "So SSSSSage, you're sssssaying one of your fellows kkkkkkilled himself over stress at work? What a tragic thing. If this were not a sssssserious topic, you know I'd have a pun. I still have one: Is this a dddead-end idea?"

Everyone groaned. Unfortunately, they would have lots of opportunities for more groaning. But that was Jonah's way of lightening things and outing his stutter. He was the elder physician in our midst, and he was my mentor. He had a way of saying things rudely yet politely. Probably the age card!

He then said the wisest thing, "The way I see this bbbbbbully thing is from the inside out. My inside to your outside."

That's when Zeke popped in and handed out the Win the Day sheet. He told everyone this was a foundation to get us all into a winning mindset. It worked well. Jonah inserted: "Good things come from the forefingers when we kkkkkeeeep them busy." We all wanted to help the team be authentic leaders, grow personally, and do both while making a positive impact.

"Precisely!" I said. "This is why when I left RHS, I started making birdhouses. For my own sanity. I needed somewhere to put the good and awful thoughts of my life and work experiences. I thought it might help us focus on the topic of bullying and where it comes from, while we have fun creating a birdhouse. My gift to you." Everyone agreed.

So, the work began.

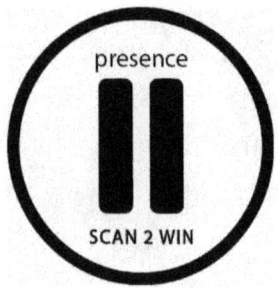

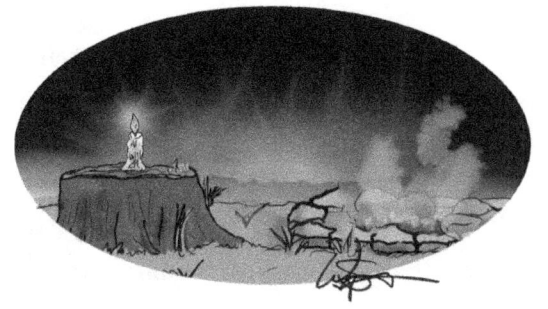

21

Burned the Candle-But Not Both Ends

Everyone

John 13:34 "Love one another."

I am only one, but still I am one. I cannot do everything, but still I can do something; and because I cannot do everything, I will not refuse to do the something that I can do.
Edward Everett Hale

Sage

Intentionally, our faces glowed in the firelight and the team started writing on the pieces of their birdhouses in between s'mores. Headlights came up the drive. It was Ananias! Only Jonah, Sarah, and now Ezekiel knew who he was to me. I introduced him, thanked him for coming, and gave him a birdhouse. He joined right in.

After about 30 minutes of deep mindful thinking, Esther was the first to speak.

Esther

I would like to share what I've written. Candy is sweet, but it doesn't mean you won't get cavities. I wrote this because it was a statement I made to a boss who really rode me and insulted me. She diminished being a professional woman to looks and skirts. She got in big trouble and lost her job, even went to jail. I gloated about it just a bit. I felt after all she'd done to me and said that she deserved it, so I gave it back to her in a quipped way. Jonah, you're right. From my inside to her outside. Isn't this like the adage about sticks and stones, but words can never hurt me?

Luke

I've scribbled: Don't patronize your partners. I wrote that because I've been called upon by many of you who were on the receiving end of bullying. I tried to reason you into resilience and placate the situation. You guys even thanked me for being the voice of reason, when all I've done is cover up your reality to get out of the uncomfortable conversation and move on. I've not been bullied, nor have I bullied anyone. At least I thought this to be true until this birdhouse mania tonight!

I have bullied others—by not being curious and recognizing their plight. I don't listen well, listening only to respond. I have built up clever things to say alongside the company line and for the greater good, but I've awakened now. I'm ignoring the greater bad. I am guilty of bystander bullying. Letting it go by like the wind, hoping it will die down. Deep inside, I expect the worst could happen to me; but, it hasn't yet. I guess I'm just tougher skinned than some. Doctor Jonah, you're on target again from inside me to the outside of others. I just put the burden back on them to do better dealing with their bullies.

Sage

We reflected.

Ezekiel raised his hand in the air. We all laughed. I asked him why he would do such a thing; we're all friends here. He said, "Well, professor I didn't want to jump in line, but I have a thought I engraved as well. May I share?"

Ezekiel

I wrote two words. It took me all this time, but here they are: Chemical Courage. I chose these because our son, Abel, has chosen a life in which he deals with his inner bully, telling him the solution is using chemical courage. The only time he can feel safe, it seems, is when he is in a bottle of gin. He will only call us when he's inebriated now, and it is in the wee morning hours. Nabal did too. I remember hearing that Nabal was difficult to deal with, and would sometimes just ramble about things that were wrong in his eyes. He had a strong sense of what works and what doesn't. He was tough on processes and easy on people, but when it came down to it, people still were afraid of interactions with him.

We tend to avoid those cries for help from one another. They don't feel warm and fuzzy. In my reluctance to face the reality of what others might be dealing with and trying to maintain that professional or authoritative parent distance, I too, like Luke, am ignoring the greater bad and don't share my authentic self.

Chemical Courage is not courage at all. It's a temporary shelter from one's authentic self, because they haven't been able to find safe shelter within or among one another.

Nabal wanted to talk to me. He left me these cards because I ditched him that night. All the things that happen in our teams seem to be driven because no one wants to or knows how to talk about it. Don't you think? Why were all those people shot to death at the ball game? Bullets aren't words, and they certainly are more powerful and permanent than sticks or stones.

Sage

We all agreed. Ezekiel was on to something.

All you could hear was the fire crackling and coyotes yipping. Beautiful brains were at work. This was important to all of us. It invigorated me and gave me hope. Then my life's hope, Sarah asked, "May I share from my viewpoint as a significant other?" Everyone tilted their heads in acknowledgment.

Sarah

I wrote one word. Be. I wrote this down because over all these years with Sage, all I could do was be. Be there with him, be for him, be through the good and the bad, be his partner over and under, in, out, you name it—I could only be. There was absolutely nothing I could do. He was doing plenty, and it wasn't working. It wasn't my place to do anything, either. As these things would come up and against him, they were also against us. We were in shock. What we lost was our ability to be. To be with one another and exist. The job became a bully that robbed us of being. We became separate. He would constantly be at work trying to fix it. He just wanted to be better. I just wanted it to be over and back to being normal.

Sage

Ruth was tearful, but added, "Yes, Sarah, to be, only to be."

Of course, through the depth of this fabulously cognitive and emotive topic came Jonah. "To bbbbBE or not to bbbbBE? That is the question!" Oh, my goodness Jonah! He sure helped break this up. There was a lot of emotion there.

Ruth

I wrote a series of words: Name it, claim it, frame it, fulfill it. This came up because I freeze when seeing bullying or being bullied. In my frozen state, I can't find any words. I get numb and I want to climb into my locker and hide like I am in middle school, hiding from the mean girls. My new husband says I'm cold and unemotional and don't talk about things. He asks me about work, and I clam up and can't talk much about it. I don't want to own my emotions. I don't know how to describe them. I rarely finish a fight. Name it, claim it, frame it, and fulfill it. I think some of this could be I don't know how to describe feelings/emotions?

Ezekiel

I don't know where to begin this. In the Army, it became my job to deliver bad news to families. Suicide news. I had to be strong in the face of this duty. It wore on me, yet I never told anyone or asked for help. I saw things. I saw things just like what Nabal did.

Ruth, that's the core of post-traumatic stress disorder. It gave me this gift of a massive heart attack. I kept pressing on like a good soldier or football star on the injured reserve list. Yet, all the while, I wasn't looking after my health or my family. Seems to me Nabal only had a few words left, and he wrote them down. These were the last ones he could muster on cards through the gin he was guzzling in his last moments.

I discount others, as I've had it tough in the military. Suck it up, buttercup, was my mantra. Now I realize that's my inner bully that drives me internally to go on for the sake of going on. I judge others that can't or won't be like me in the name of the mission.

Sage

Jonah got serious. "PPPPPplasticity. Neural plasticity and inflammation. These two are byproducts of the sssssstress you had, Zeke. No accident. You're here with that silly red heart pillow bbbbbbecause of what Ruth just told us. Ignorance is not bbbbbliss. Our bodies do keep a ssssscore ccccard on us. Nabal's mind could not pppprocess what he was thinking or ggggetting ready to dddo. He was inflamed. Inflamed with life, love, lamentation, low sssssself-esteem and lies. We must be aware and ccccurious about bbbbullying. We can wwwwin our day but shouldn't have to strive to dddddo so."

Miriam was crying and laughing simultaneously. She started, "It just kept popping up in my mind. I wanted to ignore it, but... I wrote: I love Twinkies more than I love myself or others." Ezekiel and Sarah busted out laughing, as they had heard the precious Twinkie story. Miriam continued, "I put this down because your doggie, Ruth, is adorable. But there's something about him and his name. You said one is Raja and the other Bubba?"

Ruth replied, "Yes."

Miriam said, "Years ago, a boy named Bubba destroyed our son's life."

Ezekiel interjected, "Are you sure you want to go here? Now?" Miriam said, "Yes, it is relevant, and I need to get this out. It's been buried in my heart for years. I blame him for causing all the confusion in Abel's head. He gave him traumatic brain injury. He can't reason, and he's impulsive, and Bubba did it."

Ruth commented, "My goodness."

Miriam

Ruth, your Bubba is not that Bubba, and his canine love and gorgeous big brown eyes convicted me all the while I've been scratching his ear. I must forgive this kid. He was just a kid. His mother was awful. I've made illusions in my head and heart that only Bubba could be to blame. That's not reality. I'm not present. I'm in the past, too, just like Abel. It was hockey, for crying out loud. Seems it is all Abel wants to talk about. He's stuck in the past and he uses chemical courage.

I realized that my focus has been wrong. I've been focused on the bully outside of me, not the one inside me. Doctor Jonah, you truly are a brilliant man. It is my inside pushing blaming to their outside, and they don't even know I'm having these emotions. Nor do they care. Sarah, I too have desperately wanted to just be quiet inside again. Thank you for saying that.

Sage

Jonah again provided profound prose. "Ah yes, Miriam, hurt ppppeople hurt ppppeople."

Ananias looked at me and asked, "Can I share what happened between us and why?" I nodded. I never knew why.

Ananias

I wrote exactly what Jonah just said: Hurt people hurt people. I targeted Sage something fierce and became a jailbird. He was the center of my success bullseye. I didn't like anyone older than me; but especially him. I was a young, powerful executive, and I didn't like what I was seeing in the old guard. All the while, I was never close with my father.

He was a bully of bullies. He taught me well how to be one. My father beat my mother to a pulp a few times and would tell me, "This is how you get up in the world. You beat your way to the top." Because of that, I was always results driven and trying to prove to him I was strong. Profits, not people, mattered to me. People would always get in the way of profit.

So, I railed on Sage. He was good. Too good. Sage, I'm very sorry. I was sure you would hang up on me when I called you for that reference. You didn't. One thing I didn't tell you is that my dad had cancer. It's all through his body now, and he's been dying a slow death for years.

He was a strong person. He was mean. But he got a lot of things done. My mom finally divorced him, and he was living with me because he had nowhere else to go. I had to give him his damn shots. I hated that. I would go home after work, and he would berate me. Told me I would amount to nothing, and I had to amount to something before he died, or I would be a failure. I know it's ridiculous. He was my dad. You reminded me of him. Especially when I found out about your cancer. I could not deal with you being around, reminding me of my dad and his disease.

Sage

Everyone in the group looked at me with shock on their faces. I squirmed uncomfortably, but luckily, Ananias continued.

Ananias

Rahab was pregnant. We have twin boys. I've never seen them or held them. I got what was coming to me. She turned state's evidence on me, and she got out of going to jail. I, no, we, lost a lot. I only served a few months' jail time, and we got lucky. Rahab's family helped us with a company.

It was great until I got greedy, and my eyes wandered to her best friend Hedda's beauty. Hedda and I were embezzling. I don't know why I was so driven to do wrong. Hedda told Rahab I forced myself on her and made her take the money. That was odd because the two of them schemed, and Rahab protected Hedda.

I've spent the last 10 years in prison. Funny we're making bird houses. I drew some jail bars on mine as a reminder. Thank you, Sage, for the reference. I got a job, and I'm committed to making better decisions with this third or fourth chance. And sorry if I wasn't supposed to mention that you have cancer.

Sage

There was a collective gasp at the firepit. I thought, *Jeez man, my cancer was not supposed to come up. No talk of cancer. Now what?*

Jonah saved the day. "CCCCCCancer! I cccancer see that on ya Ssssage, at all. You're the ppppicture of health!"

I had to tell them all now. "First, Ananias is right. Hurt people do hurt people. I got him fired, and I, too, like Esther, did my share of gloating. Ananias and I have buried the hatchet. We realize how this had no value for us or the organization. He got fired, and I walked away. It's why I asked him to come. Thank you, friend, for helping me get this inner bully of cancer out in the open. I'm sorry about your dad. It's not as powerful now as it was when concealed."

Sarah sighed yet agreed with me. "I am going to be, as Sarah said. Just be. I'm going to be present and curious about what time I have left and with whomever I get to spend it with. So please don't start sending flowers quite yet."

Jonah laughed. "That's a gggggggoood one Ssssage!"

Luke added, "You know, that's an important part here. I also wrote the word 'time'. Nabal must have struggled with this for a bit of time. We all have our stories, and one thing in common is time. Some let it fester, and some let it continue for time. More importantly, it was ignored at times. We passed it over, covered it up like a body in the backyard."

Jonah interjected, "Ssssslow down there, kkkkkkillller!"

"No, really, Luke is right. When bullying is ignored and not addressed, that's when our culture fails, and hurt people hurt people," I said.

Luke

I also wrote "repetitive". I chose this word because bullying is something like the scoochie koo in Miriam's Twinkie story. The bully kept on keeping on with a theme because it got a response and attention. Maybe there's another way to look at this or frame it, like Ruth said. We all know we are guilty in some way or another. Maybe instead of hiding dead bodies, we do a pulse check on each other on a repetitive basis?

Sage

Esther inquired, "Do you mean like another meeting?"

Luke said, "No, just a commitment of sorts that we will speak up when something is bugging us right then and there to help everyone win. Ruth, would that be what you're thinking fulfillment is?"

"Absolutely," said Ruth. "In Hindi there is a proverb: 'Great minds discuss ideas; medium minds discuss events; and little minds discuss people.' If we could learn to better our emotional lexicons, we'd have better words to use."

Jonah added, "Ah yes, wwwwords mmmmatter."

Luke continued, "Of course, this must be a safe place for everyone to do so, with no judgment, just curiosity, like Jonah suggested. I think of it as kind curiosity."

Miriam said, "Oh, I like that kind of curiosity." We all agreed.

"I knew you would hit this nail on its head," I said. "I've a suggestion of next steps to operationalize our thinking. Let's look at these cards, shall we? Nabal gave us two separate cards. One FOR ME and the other FOR THEM. He has a theme going here. I took the liberty of writing these on these larger boards for our eyes."

Jonah jabbed, "Sssssages Ten CCcommandments on ttttablets of wwwwood!"

"They're not mine," I responded. "They're Nabal's and now all of ours.

FOR ME

    1. Forgive me for not thinking.

    2. Forgive me for not pausing.

3. Forgive me for not talking.

4. Forgive me for not understanding.

5. Forgive me for not wanting to.

Thoughts?"

Ezekiel said, "When I saw this for the first time, deep inside, I felt a resounding 'yes and amen'. I need to first forgive myself. If I am hurt, I will hurt others. I need to stop thinking about me and me alone. I need to know who I am. Who I really am. What gets me going and what makes me go off. I need to remind myself daily what's most important. Nabal must have realized that his ways were abrasive, yet he was operating in his place of confidence."

"Good, Zeke! Good," I said. "How do we think we would become open and vulnerable to learn these things about ourselves? This is something we might need some time with to develop. It is not likely this is a magic potion. We're talking about years of background, experiences, beliefs, and habits that build each separate part of what makes up our culture."

Jonah quoted without a single stutter, "I've practiced this one for years. Edward Everette Hale once said: *'I am only one, but still I am one. I cannot do everything, but still I can do something; and because I cannot do everything, I will not refuse to do the something that I can do.'*"

I said, "The voice of wisdom rings out from Jonah again. We start with ourselves. We start by sharing our story with one another."

Luke said, "We could look at this like a bullseye. Remember that Ananias said he targeted you. Why don't we target understanding our bully tendencies? I will commit to having this drawn up in the next couple weeks. It will focus on both the helpful and not helpful outcomes of our various skills and personality preferences. I'm sure there's something already in the literature we can adopt. I think I sense two targets: one bullseye of skills, and one of emotion words to help us express, like Ruth suggested."

Sage

Everyone clapped in approval. "Thanks Luke," I said. "That is a sure start to visualize it and winning. A **Bully Bullseye.**"

Esther

Whatever we do, it's got to be easy and fun. You know, Keep it Simple Stupid. KISS. We need to have an anchor, like a brand. How about we use Sarah's 'BE' as a landing strip? There's a lot of things we can endeavor to be. Be present, be curious, be kind, be creative, be mindful, be honest, etc. Ladies, would you all join me in this one? We could get it written out, say, in a month.

Sage

Sarah, Miriam, and Ruth were all in.

Esther said, "Great! We will work on the **Beauty to BE.**"

"Okay, it's getting late," I said. "What about this FOR THEM list? Sounds like you ladies are on to something. Could this help with the BE list?"

"Yes," said Ruth. "This is in line with what Nabal wanted for us to be toward one another:

1) Get people to think about one another.

2) Get people to pause for one another.

3) Get people to talk to one another.

4) Get people to understand one another.

5) Get people to be curious enough to want to for one another."

The fire was dimming, and yawns were creeping in. We had done some heavy lifting. The big soiree was tomorrow. More people, more fun.

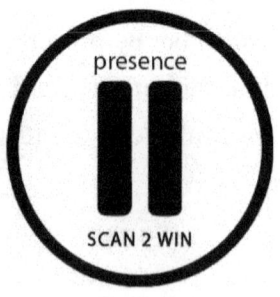

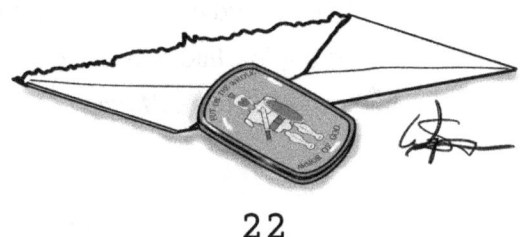

22

The Long Trip Home

Ezekiel and Ananias

Romans 15:14 "Admonish one another."

Pearl: "Challenge the status quo."

Ezekiel

Miriam and I got in the car after long goodbyes and thanks for Sage and Sarah's hospitality and love. It was time to go home. Miriam said, "You know, Sarah told me that the gent who didn't come to the gathering, Jazz, lives in the UP of Michigan. You know I've always wanted to go see Lake Superior. What do you think? Should we point our wagon north, drop by, and see if he is home?"

"Oh, Miriam. I don't have any energy to do that now," I moaned. "We're quite close to Abel. Let's go there."

"True," she said.

She tapped the GPS, and we headed for Abel's apartment. It was time to end this ghosting thing. We had to try. She called several times, and I texted, but got no answer. *Maybe he's out of town or sleeping*, I thought.

We pulled up and Miriam rustled through her purse for her address book, to see what the apartment number was. We got to the door and something in me collapsed. I wasn't sure if it was my lungs or if I was having another heart attack. I told Miriam I thought we should go and be sure he's up for a visit instead of surprising him.

She disagreed and rang the bell several more times. Nothing. I started sweating profusely. His roommate came and opened the door. "Abel, are you here?" he called out. "Your parents are here, dude."

The apartment was in full disarray. It stunk like his room. It stunk like Nabal's room. It just stunk. This whole idea stunk, and it was mine. There was Abel on the floor, behind the couch, passed out. I tried to wake him, but a bubbling white froth spilled from his mouth like a nuclear waste dump. His eyes were rolled back, and it made me dial 911.

I wiped his mouth with my hand and instinctively began CPR. I could taste the gin. The EMTs came quickly and restored his breathing. We raced behind the ambulance to the hospital. I kept blaming myself—I should have been a better father. Why did I constantly rail on him? Once Abel awoke, the first thing he said was, "I'm sorry. I need help."

We met with a social worker and the doctor, and they stabilized him. They shipped him off to an in-patient intensive rehabilitation center. We were told we could not visit for at least a week. They took Abel's phone, and he was gone. This was worse than when he was ghosting us. At least we knew he was reachable then. Now it was total silence, and not even the argumentative moments of hearing his voice and being part of what he was going through. Just solid emptiness and unknown. We knew he was there, but where?

How do you navigate this? Miriam broke down, and I held her. There was an overwhelming sense of relief, yet reluctance to believe it was finally happening. Was it too late? Is this what we all really wanted and hoped for? That was the longest week of our lives.

Abel called and told us of the withdrawals he had. He said they were better, and that he was seeing much clearer. He said, "Rehab is helping me get to know me." We were grateful and promised to visit the next week.

Miriam and Sarah kept in close contact during those few weeks. I was feeling much better and stronger, and no more coughing. I gladly dumped that beat up pillow in the trash can. Good riddance.

I felt up to a visit, so we went to see Abel at the center. It was a great time. He looked fabulous and smelled even better. He said the psychologists and neurologists were seeing him on a regular basis and it was helping. Abel wasn't blaming anyone or anything. He owned himself. He also said they were working on his resume with him to get him a job. Abel pulled me aside and said: "I'm back, Dad." Wow, it was a reality. Our prodigal had made *the long trip home*. Abel also explained a revelation he had while detoxing. He said, "Dad, in hockey I always had to win the game. I thought that was life, too. Now I win for me."

After that exhausting and exhilarating day, we headed out and Miriam brought up Jazz and the UP again. I'd been thinking about his friend, Ryder, and how they reminded me of me and Abel. We were so caught up in the visit that I never mentioned to Sage that I knew Ryder, Jazz's friend. There was an ugly separation and ghosting.

It came to me. "Miriam, I need an envelope. Do you have one?" She did. I reached in my pocket and pulled out my phone and wrote Ryder's number and name on Nabal's card labeled FOR THEM. I slipped in the "Put on the Full Armor of God," coin, wrote Jazz's address on it, and sealed it.

I told Miriam, "It would be an invasion, but I believe I have this coin for a reason. The reason Ryder gave it to me was to deliver it to restore what was broken. Maybe Jazz will get it back to Ryder." Miriam smiled. We opened the mailbox, and I deposited the envelope, pulled up the red flag and went inside.

I was tired, so I took a nap.

THE LONG TRIP HOME

The phone woke me up. It was Sarah's daughter. She delivered the news like the red flag on our mailbox. Sage was in trouble. He had been hospitalized and coughing up blood. She said the doctors didn't give him much time at all. She said Sarah could not talk nor leave his side. He was not responsive now. It was a matter of time before he took his *long trip home*. She told us not to come, but wanted us to know what was happening.

Sage passed away that evening.

I called the team to let everyone know. I sent them the obituary and funeral details. Everyone came. We knew we had marching orders to continue this work of birdhouses for bullies in his honor. Jonah did the eulogy, and I'm pretty sure he didn't have a single stutter.

Ananias asked Sarah if she would be alright if he resumed Sage's role in leading the efforts. She said, "He would like that very much."

At the funeral, Sarah handed me yet another envelope from Sage. I held it, I held her, and Miriam joined in. I knew what was in there. He would want us to complete the good work we started for Nabal and for him.

A month passed. The group put together a few tools and ideas. We decided this would be introduced at each hospital in the executive leadership teams first, and then cascaded through strategic planning retreats with all supervisors and employees.

Ananias was good at leading us. He gave us a heart-felt speech to keep the team rolling. He said, "As the weekend ended, I looked around at all of you and felt this deep sense of gratitude. Every time a bird lands on my house, I feel Sage's spirit cheering me on. You know, this experience has shown me how transformative it can be when we take the time to reflect, connect, and support each other in our growth. I know not everyone has a group like ours."

Ananias

There are programs out there, and the one that Zeke brought up, Dream Leader Institute, is a good one. I researched their website, and I'm impressed. I know we have our twist on branding towards bullying. Frankly, we identified all the good things that DLI teaches. I think we should partner with them and start helping people to win their days. We know it's never too late to create the life and leadership impact we want. I think this would honor Nabal in great fashion. In fact, Nabal's manifesto could result in us all becoming the greatest of all time in our lives sooner than we expected.

I kind of got the horse and cart in the wrong order here in these words to you, team. I took the first course in DLI. I learned about 5 choices we can make—bad, mediocre, average, really great, or world class. I made a world class decision. I went to Rahab's and knocked on the door. She opened it and at first was shocked. She nearly fainted. I reached out to catch her, and she yelled, "Don't touch me!" I told her I could say I'm sorry seven times seventy times, it wouldn't be enough. I just asked her if I could help with the twins. Her knees weakened again. She busted out crying, and said, "I love you, Ananias, you bastard!"

Yes! You see, I believe I made my *long trip home* too. This is the first world class thing I've ever done in my life.

Ezekiel

Abel had come home on Mother's Day. He and I were mowing the lawn when my phone rang. I took the call. It was Ryder. He said, "Hey, I just want you to know that my coin, (he paused and sighed) *made the long trip home*. Thanks."

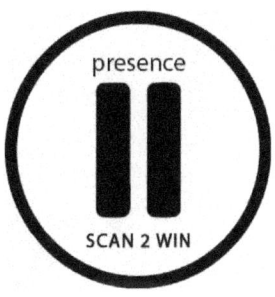

ENTITY THREE
INDIVIDUAL IMPLEMENTATION

Author's Note

Thank you for reading my book.

I promised you a three-entity book structure representing the Holy Trinity. You've now read the Intention and Insights entities. You have arrived at my final call to you. Please consider how you will individually implement and join me in:

> **Ridding the world of bullying**
> **one at a time,**
> **starting with the one in me.**

I pray it was a fun, invigorating, inspiring, and insightful reading and a thought-provoking experience for you. I trust you found time to Presence Pause while reading. My wish is that you find it useful in times of real-life need.

I hope you enjoyed the artwork, and it stimulated your curiosity. Wesley Spurgeon is a good friend of mine. He and I met when I hired him as a physical therapist. I had no idea what God had in store for us. One day he sent me a cartoon with physical therapy humor on it in an email. He asked if he could share it with our team. Of course, I was thrilled to have him encourage our team with humor. Healthcare is fun but can be serious too. When I started the book, I called Wes and asked him to do art. He obliged. Something you should know about Wes; he was an Army officer and a Blackhawk pilot. He also is an amazing wood worker. An astonishing and sad piece of Wes's life is that he has a visual challenge that is almost blinding. He draws from his heart and his fingertips. It's amazing and I'm sure it brightened your experience along the way. Thank you, Wes!

Just like the characters used birdhouses in a tangible way to process their experiences and insights, the DLI Modules provide tools and frameworks to help you identify your values, strengths, relationships, and goals. My gift to you is the Win the Day tool you just read about to get you started on this journey. Here's Wes' website: Facebook page- MaxTrq Creations.

When I was writing this book, I met Pete Van Overwalle, a professional leadership coach, who introduced me to DLI. I prayed a lot while writing, knowing I needed a powerful curriculum to combat the bully inside and the one pressing up against me externally. It was a heavenly discovery, to be honest. I became a Certified High-Performance Leader recognized by DLI and part of their mission. You can too. One thing about DLI for me was the experience of chronicling my time and how I use it. It was truly an eye-opener to see in retirement that I was a poor time manager and was missing out on my life priorities. That changed because of DLI!

I want to sincerely thank the over 70 anonymous contributors who shared their life experiences in hopes of prodding all our hearts to make ourselves and our world the greatest of all time.

AUTHOR'S NOTE

One in which humans care for one another and place others before self. One in which we start our days with a song in our hearts and a commitment to be present and to be kind.

If you will allow me just a few more words.

The Courier font you see used is not an accident. In the 1990s, I attended Northern Michigan University. I met Dr. Lon Emerick. He was a writer, and he used an old typewriter for his notes to me. They often had strike through markings. I learned so much from him about life and my professional craft. I miss him. He is the inspiration of the character Jonah. Dr. Emerick wrote me a note after grading one of my papers. I have the note on my desk, and it says:

"James, yours was the last paper I read. And the best. You write well, with a definite flair for making situations come alive. I hope you continue to hone your writing skills. (For example, keep a journal of your educational experiences). Only 10% of persons finishing an academic degree ever write anything, except perhaps publishing an article about their dissertation. ***Good things come from the forefingers when you keep them busy.***"

Most of all:

I labored and prayed over these 62,600+ words of the book. None of those moments of pondering what to write compare with the endeavor to put into words my deepest love and appreciation for my wife, Brenda, our two grown children, Brandon and Megan, and her family, Andrew, Ella, and Maya.

DREAM LEADER INSTITUTE
WIN THE DAY

DAILY REFLECTION SHEET "WIN THE MORNING AND WIN THE DAY"

My Mission Statement

My Daily Walk-Up Song

1 Word That Describes You at Your Best

5 Things I Am Grateful For

1 Thing That I Must Focus in on Today

1 Way I Can Become a Better Me Today

DREAM LEADER INSTITUTE

DREAM LEADER INSTITUTE
WIN THE DAY

DAILY REFLECTION SHEET "WIN THE MORNING AND WIN THE DAY"

5 Lies I Need to Bury Today

5 Things I Will Not Let Myself Become a Slave to Today

5 Positive Affirmations - "I Am..." (Rewrite the Narrative)

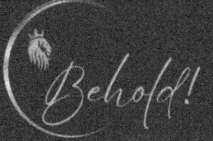

EXPLORING MY BULLY WITHIN

Professional Coaching - Speaking
James Zeigler

Ask yourself four questions below. Write your responses.
Try not to dwell on each one, just write what comes to mind first
and move on to the next question.
Authenticity is the goal here not comprehensive review.

1) How selfish am I?

2) How might my bully within be influencing my life and potential?

3) What do I admire about my bully within?

4) What do I want to say to my bully within?

Are curious about any of your responses and want to learn more? We need to talk :)

Contact me for a **FREE** Inquiry Coaching Session to chat!

906-869-1480
www.behold1.com
15440 Headquarters Rd. Tomah, WI 54660

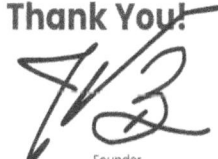

Founder

Source List

A source list is available by scanning the QR code provided below.

www.behold1.com

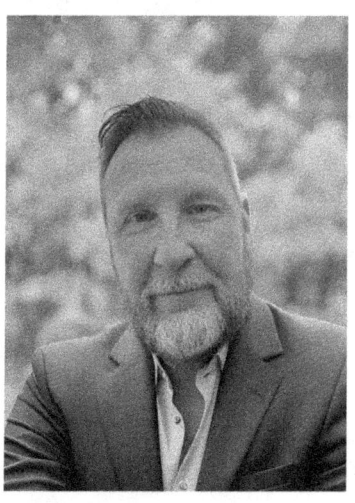

James is a husband, father, grandfather, a friend to many. He is a seasoned leader with over 35 years of experience in healthcare, specializing in helping individuals achieve a harmonious blend of leadership and life through self-awareness and the reduction of both internal and external bullying. His work focuses on empowering people to build stronger, more effective relationships, both personally and professionally, by enhancing their communication and listening skills.

Throughout his career, James has held significant leadership roles, including owner/operator of a private speech-language pathology practice, assistant professor, Chief Operating Officer, and Chief Executive Officer. He has managed organizations with operating budgets of up to $800 million and led teams of over 4,000 Full-Time Equivalent Employees (FTEE). A proud U.S. Air Force Veteran, James also served as a Senior Executive

Service Member in the Veterans Health Administration, where he contributed to shaping policy and leadership within the federal government.

As a keynote and inspirational speaker, James is passionate about guiding others to discover their full potential. His mission is simple: to equip people with the confidence to "one another," fostering kindness, collaboration, and respect. His vision is to reduce bullying by coming alongside the accusatory voice within each of us and partnering, paving the way for a safer, more compassionate world.

James is also an ordained minister, a budding author, and a lover of music. He enjoys playing guitar and writing worship music, finding inspiration in the beauty of life, faith, and service. He and his wife, Brenda have two grown children. They live in rural Wisconsin, where they cherish time with their granddaughters and bird and squirrel watching.

At his core, James believes that people are beautiful and have much to beheld—both within themselves and in the relationships they cultivate. Through coaching, he helps others discover this truth, enabling them to flourish with and for one another.

www.ingramcontent.com/pod-product-compliance
Lightning Source LLC
Chambersburg PA
CBHW020454030426
42337CB00011B/106